Help! My Child Has Cancer: My Angel On Loan

LIVING WITH A CHILD WITH CANCER

Merlon Blizzard

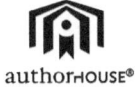

authorHOUSE®

AuthorHouse™
1663 Liberty Drive, Suite 200
Bloomington, IN 47403
www.authorhouse.com
Phone: 1-800-839-8640

First published by AuthorHouse 3/11/2009

ISBN: 978-1-4389-4285-8 (sc)
ISBN: 978-1-4389-4286-5 (hc)

Printed in the United States of America
Bloomington, Indiana

This book is printed on acid-free paper.

Contents

Dedication

This book is dedicated to the life of Asia Ariana Blizzard. The story of her life serves as a lead for the parents of children diagnosed with Neuroblastoma. Neuroblastoma is a rare childhood cancer of the sympthematic nervous system. As a mother who's lost a child to this timorous malady, I pray this message will touch others and display the guidance and knowledge that I fought to obtain. I hope for a superior study of Neuroblastoma, because it is a rare disease, and according to Sloan Kettering Memorial Cancer Center, six hundred and fifty new cases arise in the United States every year.

Questions of Life

Have you ever wondered if your life could have been different or if even the one that you are living is assigned to you to live? Perhaps the choices you've made results the way your life turned out. Life itself is a mystery and each day is a journey, yet you never know what the next day will present. Most of us walk around with an invincible mentality never thinking anything bad is going to happen. We don't have the true revelation of life. It seems some of us don't really catch on to it until we have lived almost half of our life by then its almost time to check out. Wisdom is a gift which only a few of us possesses causing us to sometimes feel misunderstood. I find that life is a puzzle and each passing day brings you the missing pieces. I realize that most people see things happening and believe it can't happen to them. People may not always have the same situations but there are a lot of similarities that we encounter. When wisdom is given to you, it feels as though you walk alone. If you are not ready it may seem life is too much to digest or comprehend, yet it is very valuable and will help you through life's times and trials. My husband often says we walk among the dead – meaning there are many that are just floating day in and day out not realizing the realities of life. My husband, a Vietnam Combat Marine, was injured and sent home with a nervous disorder, head injury, loss of hearing and Post Traumatic Stress Disorder. He sees life and war differently because traumatic situations bring different outlooks and many questions to your life. But also bring awareness to things that you never noticed. Not only did his experiences make him wiser, but also made him see life from another prospective. A great portion of his life was taken away and left him with many disabilities. The older you get the harder it is to bounce back on hard life situations.

Have you ever wondered how some people could choose to have abortions or adoptions while there are other families with children dying which they would love to keep? Have you ever thought about a funeral being a form of a message to you? While you are viewing the person's body they may be saying to you, take a good look at me because soon this will be you. That's a form of wisdom yet there are so many that never think this way. Although there are many questions, sometimes the answer is unknown while some see longevity as a blessing; some may see it as a curse. I've learned that every female is not born to be a mother whether she has children or not.

The Family Begins

As far a floating along goes, my husband and I after being married for almost four years had a daughter we named Chassity. She was quite a new experience for us, being we had never raised a child before. Most people think men are so overjoyed when they have a son, but my husband was really happy with a daughter. I believe fathers are more protective over their girls because they feel they always need a lending hand and protection. Chassity weighed eight pounds and three ounces and was a very aware child at birth. She took her little finger and held her fathers finger immediately after she was born. She seemed to have been ahead of her time during childhood, many would say she was a grown woman in a little girls body. Chassity was very particular about people and would not take to them easily. She was very careful upon whom she would associate with. Even starting day care was a task because she did not take well to strangers or even baby sitters. One baby sitter told me that Chassity would get her bottle and blanket, get on her sofa and

3

would remain content until I picked her up. She was a very cautious child, and wouldn't eat food from others. As Chassity grew older she wanted a sibling. At the age of five she asked for a sister. She seemed to be very specific. I explained to her that it takes a great amount of time and responsibility. While I thought the discussion was over she waited a while and came back again after a day of school and asked if her sister was in my stomach yet? No I said and she replied with her little boldly self "well she is going to get there because I am going to talk to God and he is going to give me my little sister". I thought to myself, "this child doesn't know what she is talking about." She then laid one of her hands on my stomach and said "God put my sister in my mother's stomach in Jesus name." I looked at her and was amazed at how much she had been paying attention in church. I admired the faith that she had. I also thought to myself that this is just a little child with desires. About a year later my husband and I became pregnant with our second child. It was amazing because I had an urge to have another child, but it was only after Chassity's request. I often wondered about that prayer and began to look at Chassity in a different manner. Now it was time to tell Chassity the news. When informed she said "I know it's my sister", I said lets wait and see. She said I don't have to I wait I know it's my sister because I asked for her. By this time Chassity was in first grade. What an experience she was because she was excited about riding the

4

school bus but soon was ready to quit school. She possessed a great attachment to us and her grandmother and did not cope well with separation from us. Eventually she decided at the age of six she was finished with school. I recall times when I would leave her at home for her father to take her to school, I would call to see how things went and she would be at home with her dad because when they'd arrive at the school and she would cry and run back grabbing his legs therefore dad could not stand to leave her. I guess my husband hated to see her cry. The teacher sensed the attachment and recommended for her to try the bus. After a few weeks she finally adapted. Three months later I had an ultrasound. I informed Chassity and she said she already knew it would be a girl. I told Chassity lets pray that the baby is in the right position so that we would see the sex of our child and sure enough it was a girl. Chassity wasn't worried because she had the faith of a mustard seed and she knew for sure her prayer was answered. As time progressed I begin to feel the urge to prepare my baby's nest. I began to clean, prepare the baby's bag and pack my bag for the hospital. This is nature's way of letting the mother know that the baby is coming. I had gone to the doctor and was told that I had started dilating. I felt very tired when I came home from work so after cooking for my family I laid down. I remember it was a Friday night and I dosed off to sleep. I was awakened by my water breaking. Chassity was lying beside me in bed as I started shouting "my water has broken." I told my husband it was time to go to the hospital and it seemed the water continued to flow until I arrived at the hospital. It seemed as my husband was driving the bumps in the road made the pain worse. The pain was excruciating and very intense. When I arrived at the emergency room my dress was soaked. They thought I was ready for delivery; however it was four more hours before she arrived. It felt like when I was pushing the insides of my head was coming out as well. I asked for pain medication and an epidural but the doctor said no because my labor was moving along very well so I felt everything. Our new little girl arrived November 4th 1995 weighting seven pounds and fifteen ounces, both girls were twenty and a half inches long. We named her Asia Ariana (meaning angel). My husband and Chassity were both present as Asia's birth and the nurse told Chassity that Asia looked just like her.

Asia Comes Home

As I was released from the hospital we went home to adapt to our new addition to the family. As it seemed Asia developed a lot of gas from drinking the milk. She began to cry as I would try to make her burp more hoping to relieve the gas. As a result of this we carried her to the doctor and he said that some babies have trouble digesting milk and prescribed a different milk formula. I also noticed that at times when Asia did burp a lot of milk would come out of her mouth. The doctor then told me to use Mylicon drops for her gas. When I tried to breast feed her she disliked that, I guess it's because she started off with the bottle. Asia also seemed to be ahead of her time. She too was a grown woman in a little girl's body. Asia seemed to be like any ordinary child, happy, playful and very choosy about people. She developed as a normal child would and looked so much like Chassity and everybody thought they looked like twins. Asia still continued to still have problems digesting her milk causing her formula to be changed several times. Besides her digesting problems

7

she seemed to be a happy child. We took lots of pictures and videos as they were growing up. These were treasured years and moments that we only get to experience once. Time seemed to be moving fast as my busy schedule required me to work and take care of a husband and two girls. There was always something to do and not enough time to do it. Taking care of two children was very difficult but they were truly treasured gifts from God.

A Minor Limp

Time has gone past and now Chassity is now nine years old and
Asia was three years old. Asia begun to limp as she walked and also
began to demand being held. She told us that her leg was hurting
so we took her to the doctor. During the visit the doctor asked if
she had fallen, we could not recall her falling but toddlers are busy at
that stage of life. After the doctor x-rayed her leg the doctor told us
that he found nothing wrong. We left the doctors office, but still paid
close attention to her to see if she would get better. I still continued
to give her children's Tylenol for pain. The limp became so intense
that she got to the point that she needed to be carried more. She then
told me that her arm was in pain and she developed a sudden fever.
We carried her back to the doctor's office and told him about her leg
and arm and the increasing disability with her walk. The doctor again
stated that the previous x-ray proved that nothing was wrong with
her. I replied that a child does not limp for no reason at all and that
there is something wrong. I also told him that I was still giving her

9

Children's Tylenol for pain and fever. I then demanded for a re-x-ray

of her leg and also her arm which she was complaining about. He did

the x-rays and then drew blood and then told us that we would have

to go to the Children's Hospital of the Kings Daughters in Norfolk,

Virginia. Her hemoglobin was very low and he referred us to the

Hematology clinic because he suspected she had Leukemia. As tears

began to run down my face I looked at the doctor and said" you must

have made a mistake, my child does not have Leukemia". I knew the

word Leukemia meant cancer and like anyone else I never imagined

this happening to me. The doctor sent the x-rays over to the hospital

and told us they would discuss the results of the x-rays upon our

appointment at the Hematology clinic.

As we walked into the Hematology clinic at the hospital of the

Children's Hospital of the Kings Daughters I questioned my reason

for being there. A doctor called Asia's name and asked if I knew why

we were there. I said I was referred by Asia's pediatrician because he

suspects she may have Leukemia. He insisted on taking blood test

and mentioned that he suspected she had Neuroblastoma. I asked

him what that was. The doctor said lets do some test first before

discussing it. The blood work came back negative for Leukemia but

further testing was needed to understand why her blood level was

so low. He said either her body was not producing red blood cells or something was taking them away. By this time another doctor came in to review her x-rays while examining he discovered a tumor was lying behind her pelvic. He had to do more testing to find out what type of tumor it was. More doctors entered the room and begin to press on her pelvic area. "There it is "the doctor said, another doctor touched the same area for accuracy. He told us the tumor was located behind her pelvic bone and to detect the type of tumor some tissue would have to be removed. Little Asia was transferred to the operating room for a biopsy and a bone marrow aspiration. My husband and I sat in the waiting room with harsh devastation desperate to know what is going on with our daughter. This was the first time we had ever heard of Neuroblastoma. After the surgery we were called in a room where we were informed that the illness was in fact Neuroblastoma. We were more devastated now because we had never heard of this illness. January 1999 Asia was admitted to the hospital. More testing such as cat scans, bone scans, and MRI were performed. After the entire test was completed the doctor brought the scan films into her room so that we could view them. There were tumors from her head to her feet including two large tumors an inch from her spinal cord and one behind her pelvic area. The doctor stated if she would have went much longer she would have been paralyzed for life. We both felt as though we could fall through the floors. He then mentioned that Neuroblastoma is life threatening and does not have many survivals. He also stated her prognosis was very poor. We began asking many questions such as what can be done and requested a specialist for this type of cancer.

Neuroblastoma is a form of cancer that occurs in infancy, childhood and some adults. The cells of the cancer resemble developing nerve cells found in the embryo or the fetus. The term neuron indicates "nerves" while blastoma refers to cancer that affects immature or developing cells. These cells are essential for our thinking, sensation, and movement. It usually starts in the adrenal glands sympthamatic nervous system or among the chest, pelvis and neck. Neuroblastoma is the second most common type of solid tumor in children. The disease affects one out of eighty thousand to one hundred thousand children under the age of fifteen each year. Nearly ninety percent of cases are diagnosed at age six. There are no avoidable risk factors for neuroblastoma and there are no know ways to prevent the disease. Screening for Neuroblastoma will result in earlier diagnosis and better treatment results. Results show that screening infants at six months does increase the number of cases in Neuroblastoma found in which you will see that it is not being done due to the reason many experts feel that screening will not lead to decrease from death in Neuroblastoma in which I argue the difference because the earlier the state of cancer the better the survival rate will be and can be treated effectively.

However, in many cases the disease is not diagnosed until it has already metastasized (spread). The most common signs of Neuroblastoma are an unusual lump or mass that is found in the child's abdomen causing it to swell, abdominal fullness, discomfort, or pain. Masses can occur in other places and can spread to the back of the eye causing it to protrude and if metastasis to the bones has occurred a child who can walk may complain of bone pain which causes the child to limp, refuses to walk or is unable to walk. Pressure on other nerves near the spine can cause the child to lose the ability to move the arms or legs and blue or purple patches may indicate spread to the skin. If the bone marrow is affected the child may not have enough red blood cells, white blood cells, or blood platelets which can result in weakness, frequent infections and excessive bleeding from small cuts or scrapes. In about ninety percent of cases Neuroblastoma cells can be detected by a test for neurotransmitters called catecholamine in blood or urine samples.

The doctor went on to say that Asia had a twenty percent survival rate and that she was at stage 4 of the disease which is very fatal and the last stage of her cancer. I began to wonder why is this happening to me and my family. I began to have many questions for God. The doctor informed us about a hospital in New York that specialized in Neuroblastoma cancer; we told him we would be interested in talking with them before any treatment was started. The doctor went on to say that Neuroblastoma cancer is usually treated with very high and

heavy doses of chemotherapy, radiation and a possible bone marrow

transplant; however the Children's hospital of Kings Daughters did

not do transplants. The doctor contacted the sources in New York

in order to have a conversation with them while my husband was

speaking to the physician his facial expressions were looking very

dim and disturbed. I could tell that he wasn't hearing good news. I

was introduced to a lady that had a child with the same type cancer,

her child the same age as Asia and she spoke about the treatment

at the hospital in New York. She was such a help to me because I

knew nothing about Neuroblastoma and the impact it would have

on our lives. She told me that she rented her house out and stayed in

New York for her child to receive treatment. While she was talking

to me, I was still in shock so some of it didn't register at that time.

I still think her Pediatrician missed her disease at an earlier state

because according to her problems with the digestion of milk and the

first time we carried her in about her limp these were symptoms of

Neuroblastoma.

The First Stage of Treatment

The conversation still did not entail everything this disease would entail. After consultation with the physician in New York we decided to go with Sloan Kettering Memorial Hospital treatment plan, so they prescribed the N7 Protocol which included seven to eight courses of high dose chemotherapy plus surgical resection of bulk disease. Courses 1,2,4,6 consisted of 6 hour intravenous infusions of cyclophosphamide on days 1 and 2, a 72 hour intravenous infusion of doxorubicin and vincristine beginning day 1, and vincristine bolus on day 9. Courses 3, 5, and 7 consisted of 2- hour intravenous infusions of VP-16 on day's 1 to 3 and 1 hour intravenous infusions of Cisplatin on day's 1 to 4. Courses were to start after neurotfil counts reach 500microL and platelet counts reached 100.000 micro. Vincristine which is a white liquid and is given through the vein and the common side effects are drooping of the eye lids, blurred or double vision, jaw pain, seizures, constipation, stomach pain, hair loss and irritation of the nerves, numbness and tingling of fingers and toes, muscle weakness and Doxorubicin which is red liquid that is administered through the vein and the side effects are nausea/vomiting, hair loss, urine may turn pink/red for one to two days after treatment, low blood counts one to two weeks after treatment, mouth sores, heart damage, nail beds may change color and texture and the skin may be more sensitive to sunlight in the areas of the body which have received radiation therapy. Heart test are done before this drug is given and certain times throughout the course of treatment to check heart function. This medication can be irritating to the tissue if it leaks out of the vein. Etoposide (VP-16) is also a clear liquid and is given intravenously and the side effects are nauseated/vomiting, loss of appetite, hair loss, low blood counts, mouth sores, low blood pressure, fatigue, abnormal liver function tests and allergic reactions. Cisplatin is a clear liquid given through the vein (IV) and the side effects are nausea/vomiting, loss of appetite, hearing loss, most often in higher tones, kidney damage, low blood counts, low level of magnesium in the blood, numbness and tingling in fingers and toes, allergic reactions and seizures. Cisplatin can also cause kidney damage and blood test is done frequently to check the minerals, especially magnesium in the blood. A hearing test is done after receiving this treatment and at certain times during treatment monitoring the kidneys. Cytoxan is a clear liquid that is given (IV) intravenous and the side effects are nausea/vomiting, loss of appetite, hair loss, and low blood counts one to two weeks after treatment, blood in urine, metal taste in mouth, hormonal changes and heart damage with high doses. This medication can also cause bladder irritation and a medication called mesna is given along with this chemotherapy to help prevent bladder irritation. Intravenous fluids are used heavily to help push the chemotherapy out of the body to help with the bladder. Now before her chemotherapy could be started she had to have a central venous line inserted in her chest which is a long hollow tube made from silicone rubber which is inserted (tunneled) under the skin of the chest into a vein. The tip of the tube sits in a large vein just above the heart. The space in the middle of the tube is called a lumen. Sometimes the tube has two or three lumens. At the end of the tube outside the body each lumen has a special cap to which a drip line or a syringe can be attached. There is also a clamp to keep the tubes closes when not being used. The central line was inserted for chemotherapy, antibiotics and intravenous fluids. It was also used to take samples of blood for testing and to give liquid food if her digestive system was not able to cope. This made treatment possible without having to inject needles in her veins. The central line was inserted by cutting the skin near her collar bone; the tip of the tube was threaded in a large vein under anesthesia. Afterwards, a chest x-ray was performed to insure that the tube was in the correct place. It was then covered with dressings, and she was given pain medications for the soreness and discomfort. The tissue under the skin grew around the cuff in about three weeks and held the line safely in place but until then stitches held it into place. We learned that hubby and I had to be trained to care for the central line because it would be used frequently and required special care to prevent Asia from getting infections, also to prevent blockage in the lines. A small amount of fluid (Heparin) had to be pushed through the lines weekly or after any medication was administered to keep the lines from getting blocked. The site of where the lines were placed had to be given a sterile dressing twice a week to reduce the risk of infection. This was not easy to do to my own child, especially when you had to see the hole where the line entered. No air was allowed to get into the lines and we had to be sure that the line was not cut or broken. After setting up the protocol with the Children's Hospital of Kings Daughters, and three chemotherapy treatments were completed, we were to report to Sloan Kettering Memorial Hospital in Manhattan, New York for further treatment. It was now Feb 2, 1999 and Asia would be starting her first chemotherapy treatment in which she had to receive pre-medication such as Zofran to help prevent nausea, Decadron was used to help kill some cancer cells and increase the effectiveness of the other anti-cancer drug, mesna was used to help prevent the bladder from being irritated and finally chemotherapy began. She was an in-patient since we decided to have her first three chemotherapies at our local hospital. They started the chemotherapy at night because they felt it was better for the child to try and sleep through it. Seventy two hours seemed long to me for chemotherapy. As the chemo bag began to drip, Asia was receiving chemotherapy for the first time; we did not know what to expect other than the loss of her hair. She started showing the results of the chemotherapy very quickly as her hair begin to loosen from her scalp. She also began to get sores in her mouth as well as her eye brows and eye lashes disappeared. It was very painful to watch what the drugs were doing although they were killing cancer cells as well as her good cells. After the chemotherapy was finished being administered the doctors told us that her immune system would drop completely and she would develop fever and if the fever gets to 101 we'd have to bring her back immediately to the hospital because her immune system would be gone and she would develop infection which could result in death. Sure enough she developed a fever and we were back at the hospital in about three or four days. Her blood counts dropped dramatically. Her Neutrogena (white blood cells) was low and she was put into isolation until her blood cells came back up. After chemotherapy she was given a medication named (neuroses), which helps speed up the growth of white blood cells in the bone marrow. The white blood cells are called Europhiles which help fight infection. Neuroses were given every day by the use of a needle inserted into her skin until her white blood cell count increased. This was extremely painful for her and us because she would cry when she saw the needle. Just imagine your three year old having to look forward to this for ten to fourteen days. Each time she received chemotherapy it would take longer for her immune system to bounce back. We were also trained to give her shots. When we took her home we would have to give them to her. I hated sticking a needle in her skin and watching her cry. When it was time to give them to her at home the whole house was disrupted because everyone in the whole house was torn to threads. We asked if there was a way she could be given the neupogen intravenously and the doctor said the medication was more effective with needle injection. However I do believe some kids are receiving it now intravenously. We had to draw her blood from her central venous line, ((broviac) to carry to the hospital to check her blood counts. We were given some Emla cream used to numb the area for the injection. Neupogen came in a box of ten very small vials and for a box of ten, it cost twelve hundred dollars and Asia began to use over ten vials in order for her white blood cells to recover. She also had to be intravenously fed because of the sores in her mouth; the metal taste caused a loss of appetite as well. The chemotherapy hit her little body really hard so we were in the hospital for over a month waiting for her to bounce back. I then contacted my employer again to request time off due to family illness. I also applied for family medical leave because I did not know when I would be returning back to work at this point because as soon as her blood counts would return if would be time for her next cycle of chemotherapy. Our whole lives were changed and we also had Chassity to consider making sure she could get to school, help her with her homework and still make ways to travel with Asia. My mother assisted me with Chassity and a family dog that we had to make arrangements for as well. While being at the local hospital I would stay with Asia while hubby would take care of the errands. But going to New York would be a different adventure to deal with. While Asia was in the hospital, she was treated with a variety of antibiotics to prevent her from developing infections. After being released from the hospital, it would be time for chemotherapy again in two weeks. In between the hospital stays, we had to take Asia to the hematology clinic to have her blood counts checked on a regular basis two to three times a week meant long days at the clinic. Her blood counts determined if she needed platelets or blood transfusions. It would take four to six hours to receive her blood intravenously and then platelets depending which one the hospital would receive first. Now that her counts are back up Asia begin to bounce back. Time was approaching for the second chemotherapy treatment. It seemed as soon as your child was feeling better it was time to knock them back down again. Asia seemed to adapt well with her hair being gone

and never complained about it. She was really happy to have all three
of us with her. Chassity was like a miraculous medicine for Asia. She
always seemed to light up when she had Chassity with her. Chassity
would get in the bed with her, they were very close.

Back for Asia's chemotherapy, another four to five hospital stays
for the administration. Once again we were released to go home and
told to watch for fevers. Sure enough we were back at the hospital
again. Asia once again begins to develop a high fever, her immune
system dropped and antibiotics had to be used to reduce infection
and prevent death. Due to the immune system being so low she
did not have enough white blood cells to fight off the infection. We
had to stay until the blood counts were up so this was another long
hospital stay. We began to notice our finances depreciating while
wondering about the life of our child as well. After we were released
from this chemotherapy treatment we had to once again take her
back to hematology clinic for the checking of her blood counts and
this would determine her next chemotherapy treatment. While I
was at the hospital during Asia's second chemo my pastor called and
asked me to bring Asia to church for prayer. I said I would if she was
able to come. It would depend on her blood counts. He said that
if we could not bring her, then send a picture to hold for prayer. I
started praying and asking God to help me with Asia with the prayer

service. Sure enough we were able to take her to the prayer service
and she received her special prayer. After coming home from Asia's
second chemotherapy treatment, she was sitting on the floor playing
in the den and as I was watching her she began starring at something.
I called her name several times, but she continued to stare. I then
called her name again and she responded. I asked her what was
she looking at? She said "Mama didn't you see it?" I said to her see
what? She said "the angel," she said "she was standing right there." I
then asked her what did she look like? She said the angel had on all
white and was very pretty. The way she was starring I knew she was
really looking at something. It was time for the third chemotherapy
and for another four to five days we had to watch our little girl get
hooked up to the intravenous lines for chemo which moved slowly
throughout her vein, while we watched for side effects. We began
to take video tapes for her to watch to help her through her stays.
When she felt like it we would play games with her. The hospital
had a play room that she could attend if she didn't have low blood
counts. Once again we had gotten through another chemotherapy
treatment and were released to go home. It really made us appreciate
freedom, because staying in the hospital was like a form of prison
when you have to constantly stay there. Again we are traveling back
and forth to the Children's Hospital for the checking of Asia's blood
counts and for transfusions of blood and platelets. This went on

for about a month. Each time that she received a chemotherapy treatment it took her longer for her blood counts to come back to normal. This showed that chemotherapy was taking a great effect on her body. As we were on our way back home from the hematology clinic we stopped at the seven eleven store. My husband went in to get us some goodies to eat. Asia asked me to read her Pinocchio book in which she received from the hospital. I started reading the book to her on our way home. After about one hour of riding home still reading to Asia as I was reading to her a picture of an angel was in the book and she said to me "it resembled the one I saw". I thought she must be really seeing this angel. She assured me that she did see this angel. One of the families that I met that also had a son diagnosed with Neuroblastoma shared a story with me about their son talking to someone in his bedroom when they asked him who was he talking to he told them there were some angels talking to him and telling him to come and go with them. He told them not right now he needed to stay with his mother.

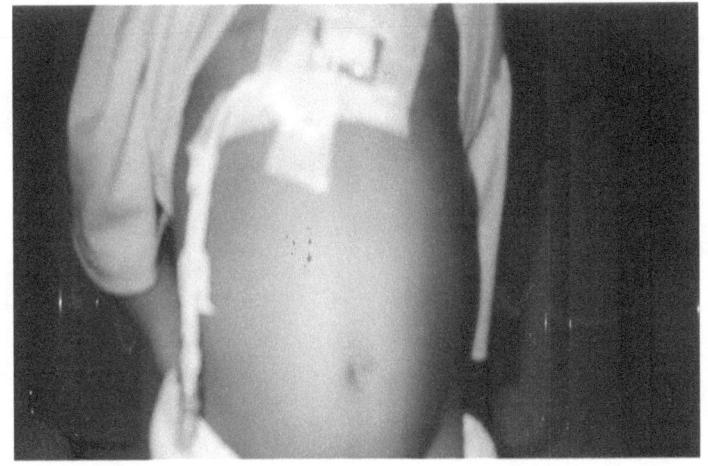

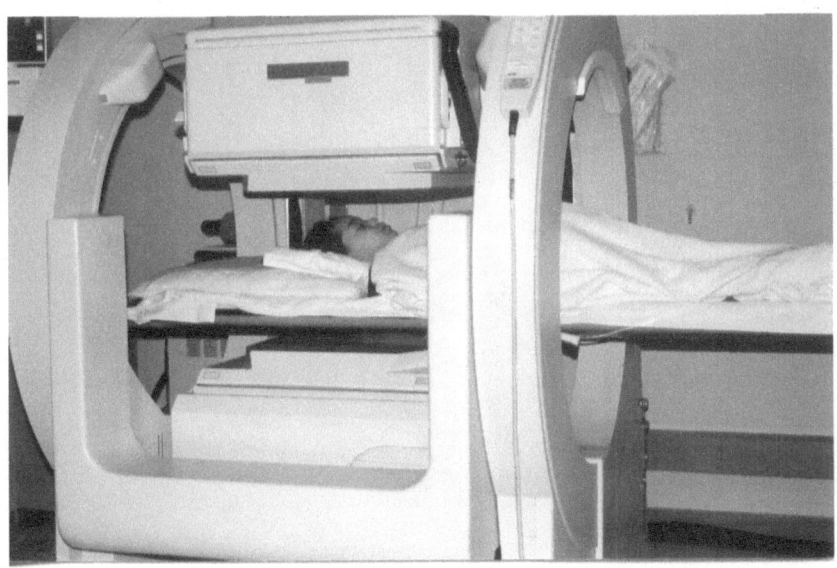

Our First Chemo in New York

Now that she is ready for chemotherapy it is time to go to New York to see the specialist to see how well she had responded to her chemotherapy treatments. We are now wondering how we were going to get to New York and questioning about arrangements for Chassity and the dog. Of course we are thinking about driving but wondering where we were going to stay not knowing how long we would be there. The hospital social worker called us to inquire about our traveling arrangements and if we had things set up to come. I told her we were considering driving because it was cheaper than flying but she told me that parking would be very difficult and expensive. She said to garage our vehicle would cost at least fifty dollars a day. She suggested flying to prevent the parking problem and asked if we would be interested in staying at the Ronald McDonald House. She went on to explain how the Ronald McDonald House operates and that she could make arrangements to set up a room for us. She told us to notify her when we arrived at the

Ronald McDonald House and that they would notify her. She stated she knew how the situation would impact our family and that most families didn't know what to expect when they arrived. She was such a blessing to our lives as we were walking so much in the darkness of this disease and what was happening to us. I made arrangements for Chassity to stay with my mother. She would be helping Chassity get to school and looking out for her. We left our pet dog with my husband's best friend which was like a brother to him. We booked our flights to Manhattan, New York for Asia's first appointment. We had to also make arrangements to get from our home to the airport which meant have someone pick up our vehicle from the airport. Of course we had to go through the line at the airport for our tickets which didn't go smoothly, dealing with the crowds and luggage was a hassle, only able to have two bags and a stroller as well. In New York you do a lot of walking. Asia could not always walk the whole way to the hospital. As soon as we arrived to the Big Apple the first thing we noticed was the different cultures and an enormous population of people. New York is different from Virginia in many ways. Manhattan is so much more convenient. Everything you need is so handy and available. You really don't need a car to live there because the subways, the buses, taxicabs and your very own legs will carry you anywhere you need to go. You have no traveling problems there and it's much cheaper to travel. You just stand out on the corner of the street and hold out your arm to flag the cab down. Of course

they also drive there like they are crazy. Don't get in their way or

you will be sorry. Even on the subway and the buses if you don't get

on quick you may get shut up in the door. The pace is much faster

and people are really on the go there. It's hard to walk the streets

without touching someone. In some parts of New York you should

not wear your jewelry showing or it may get snatched off before you

know it. They seem to have newer technology there and are a lot

more advanced. Now that we have arrived in New York we had to go

through the airport to obtain our luggage and get a taxicab to carry us

to the Ronald McDonald House.

A Home Away From Home

The first Ronald McDonald House was established in 1974 in Philadelphia, Pennsylvania. It has extended over a period of time in various locations. I stayed at the Ronald McDonald House funded from charities. The Ronald McDonald House is a home away from home for families undergoing cancer treatment. Standing eleven floors high, it holds eighty-three families. The capacity of the building is usually always full. The building starts at the basement which has a playroom, the Giants playroom, game room and computer center. The first floor is where the foyer is located as well as the living room, library, board room and the Chapel. The second floor has a dining floor and kitchen that is assigned to each room. The third floor is known for the Terrace and the ninth floor is known for the sun room. All of the other floors are for families with children with cancer. It helps approximately twelve major cancer centers, which makes it easier for families to get treatment on a regular basis. At that time if you could financially afford it you were charged thirty five dollars a night. Children come from all over the

world to the Ronald McDonald House for cancer treatment. A lot of

people bonding are taken place once you enter it because everyone is

fighting the same battle so everyone can relate to each other. You can

look into the eyes of people and feel the connection. They offer arts

and crafts, cooking; give a ways, dinners, breakfast, pizza and movie

night as well as entertainment and parties. They seem to understand

what the families are going through knowing that the time you share

there will soon be coming to an end. You get to know a lot of their

staff and volunteers because you stay there for long periods of time.

You see so much sickness, along with your own trial that it changes

your whole concept of life itself. The children that visit seem to

relate very well to each other because they see that it is a lot of them

living in a different world from kids that aren't sick. The Ronald

McDonald House is a big help with helping children through their

treatment. They always have something to offer to make a child smile.

They keep them occupied so that it doesn't seem that they are just

living in a hospital. They have something to look forward to as they

approach their treatment days. They celebrate all the holidays so

even though you are not at home you don't have to miss Christmas,

Easter, Thanksgiving or your birthday. If they know your birthday

is coming they give you a party and gifts. When we finally arrived at

our home away from home we tried to unwind from all the traveling hassles of getting there and trying to prepare ourselves for what was to come. The night passed and morning came as we were getting ready to go to the hospital for our next adventure. The hospital is rated the number one cancer center in the world. We walked there from the Ronald McDonald House. It was June 1999, the weather was a little warm but the walking was good for us. We met the doctors whom we had been communicating with for the last three or four months, they told us they needed to do a bone marrow aspiration test to see the status of the cancer in order to decide if surgery was needed. The test was done and surgery was needed to remove some tumors and her adrenal gland. We met with the surgeon whom is known to be able to remove tumors that other physicians would not do. We discussed the procedure and set the date for surgery. Asia had to be prepped, meaning a tube had to be administered through her nose to dispense liquid that would allow her body to cleanse itself. She could only have Jell-O or water the night before. It was painful watching them put the tube down my little girl's nose, knowing they were going to cut my baby. It was harder because she could not make any of the decisions on her own. Every decision was left up to me and her father. I can still feel the pain pierce the inside of me as I write this. I felt so helpless and wished it would just all go away. The hospital rooms were very small and there is very little space. There is a curtain between you and another child sharing a room. It seemed like one of the longest nights yet not in a hurry to see tomorrow either. Dad and

I stayed with her as they had recliners that made it suitable to stay

with your child. The hospital seemed to understand family neediness

with these life threatening situations. They knew that our days with

our children were very precious moments to us and understood that

healing was more effected when the children were surrounded with

their love ones. The hospital is twenty one stories high and was filled

with adults and children who are fighting cancer. I saw people with all

different types of cancer and although they say Neuroblastoma is rare

it did not look rare there. The hospital was constantly receiving new

patients; I saw newborns with chemotherapy running though their

veins. I saw many sad faces and tears running down parents faces. As

we would come and go, we heard about children that we constantly

saw had passed on.

Morning had arrived and it was time for Asia to be taken in for

surgery. They put her to sleep before they moved her from us. As

they rolled her into the operating room, tears began to roll down my

cheeks. My inner being was filled with pain and sadness believing

God would bring her back to me. So now her dad and I waited

for her to come from surgery in the lounge which seemed so hard.

Thoughts were just running through our minds. There were other

people in the lounge as well waiting for their love ones to return from surgery. You could hear some of the reports and the news wasn't sounding good. I got up to go to the bathroom to cry and pray "Lord please let my little girl come back to us". The waiting room was filled with sadness. After about five hours we received a phone call from the receptionist desk telling us Asia had been taken to recovery and as soon as she was situated we would be allowed to see her. The doctor told my husband he was amazed at her response to the chemotherapy that she had taken. He said a lot of the tumors had shrinked tremendously. I immediately thought about the special prayer done for her at church and of all the people that was praying for her.

As Asia became situated from recovery, we could go in and see her. I was so happy just to be close to her. She was still sleep with tubes in her arms and down her nose. She was very swollen as the doctor said that came from the surgery. After this, she was taken to intensive care to another hospital through a tunnel that runs across the street. She opened her eyes at this point and looked at me. I said to her "I am right here as I told you I would be when you wake up". She was given morphine for pain. We sat with her all night in intensive care. The hospital had lounge chairs, so if we needed to lie down, we could go to a lounge room down the hall. Asia was out most of the night while they tried to keep her comfortable. Asia was cut from under her breast bone down to her lower abdomen area. It hurt tremendously to see my child in that condition, thinking all that she had gone through to survive. The next day Asia was still out of it , so we sat with here until about one o'clock in the morning, then decided to go down to the lounge. Dad and I were really worn and stressed out. Before I went, I told Asia to tell the nurse to come get me if she needed me earlier. During that morning Asia woke up and asked the nurse for me. I came to her bedside (dad along) and Asia told me that she pulled the tubes out of her nose. I thought the morphine that had been given to her was just talking, but the nurse replied "she sure did and she does not need them put back". Asia then said "mama I want to get in your lap". I thought what a soldier. The nurse was standing by and told Asia to let her give her some medicine and then they'd try and let her get into my lap. The nurse and dad assisted her into my lap. It was like an unreal feeling just to hold my child. I had such a joy inside of me but tears at the same time. After she was in my lap for a little while I think she started feeling uncomfortable, she was ready to get back in the bed and was given more morphine for pain. The next day the nurse mentioned that she was responding well and that she'd be released to a regular hospital room. The nurse said we call her a flying patient, because it was unusual how she flew right in and out. She thought her recovery was fast. Once again I thought about prayers being answered. When Asia was moved from intensive care unit to a regular hospital room we were moving right along. The next day the doctor came in and told us that as soon as she sits up she can be discharged, but she'd need chemotherapy again and then they'd determine when she could go home. So we began to ask Asia how bad did she want to get out of the hospital and she tried to sit up. I told her that if she works with her dad whom was helping her to sit up we could leave the hospital and go back to the Ronald McDonald House. It was painful for her but dad got her to sit up and put her in her stroller. The doctor came back the next day and permitted that she could leave. So off to the Ronald McDonald House we went. This was all such a hard and stressful thing to do, it still hurts.

The following chemotherapy was to start at seven o'clock the next morning. There were not a lot of breaks in between treatments as they explained to us that Neuroblastoma is not the type of cancer that you give time to grow. They explained it as if you were fighting a war and when you go in to kill the enemy you must kill them all because if one is left, it can destroy everything. Just one cell could start up another whole army. At Sloan Kettering, chemotherapy was done as an outpatient; we had to arrive very early because we'd be there all day and possibly to seven or eight at night, only to return again the next morning. She was sent to the Ronald McDonald house with an IV bag hooked into her line which ran all night till the next morning. It helped flush the chemo to be ready to start again the next morning.

The treatment was very aggressive and intensive. After finishing this cycle of chemo, the doctor told us that we could return to Virginia, but we had to return to the local hospital for blood platelets. There were no breaks because we were at Children's Hospital of Kings Daughters at least three times a week and the days were very long. By this time our newly changed lives and our finances were very low and things were getting further and further behind. We started inquiring about help services that may be available to us. The social worker in New York told us about the American Cancer Society and the Cancer Care society who assist families but the services are limited due to the volume of people in need. The American Cancer Society assisted a one time house payment but they could not continue to help with our mortgage payments. We were continuing to get behind on all our bills as well as money needed to travel back and forth for Asia's treatment. The list goes on plus medical bills were adding us as well. Traveling and living in two places was very expensive. I began to ask for leave donations from my job to see if I could obtain some monies to help out. I needed more than anything to be able to stay with my child.

After Asia's counts came back to normal we had two more chemotherapy treatments at our local hospital and it would be time to return to Sloan Kettering in New York again. Now our trips

were longer and more frequent with the treatments to come. This
time after our last chemo on the protocol, the doctors at Sloan
Kettering did another bone marrow test on Asia and told us that
she was in remission. That news was better than gold because with
this disease, most children never see remission. Although the doctor
felt she was in remission, he recommended that we should do one
more chemotherapy. Once again it was an early morning, leaving
the Ronald McDonald House around seven o'clock in the morning
and getting back about six or seven at night. Chemo ran through
her veins all day and IV fluid bag was to run all night. This would
be going on for three to four days. Once this chemo was over we'd
have to go to the clinic every other day for blood counts, platelet
checks, and transfusions when needed. They were needed because
the chemotherapy doses always took her blood counts down and we'd
have to be very cautious about infections because of her immune
system. After her counts returned to normal, we'd have to look
forward to radiation treatment and a bone marrow transplant. You
think when you hear the word remission you think you are safe, but
you find out you still have quite a ways to go with this disease. After
each chemotherapy treatment we would have to wait until Asia was
ready to eat as her taste buds changed. She would only eat certain
foods. We tried to get her to eat whatever she would, because chemo
takes your appetite as well. Radiation would be to her chest and

pelvic area. It consisted of about fifteen days, but first the sites of radiation had to be marked in order to display her body would receive the radiation. Still in New York, having the radiation done meant she would feel tired and could possibly feel nauseous after the radiation sessions so when we went to get radiation, she would have to be put on the table and she would have to lie very still. If she couldn't stay still, they'd have to pt her under anesthesia. She did not want to be put to sleep, so she laid still and we'd walk out the door. We could see her and talk to her through a glass window which helped her go through the procedure. Asia did not like to be left alone and as long as she knew we were close by, she would do her treatment. Before the bone marrow transplant could be performed, a portion of her bone marrow is extracted from her and is destroyed as a result of high dosage of chemotherapies and radiation, so it is harvested and frozen, then placed into storage until usage. Bone marrow is harvested by using needles and syringes to draw out a large amount of the marrow from the hip bones under anesthesia. Processing of the marrow might include cleaning it with the drug called 3F8 which can kill tumor cells in harvested bone marrow and can be later given back to the patient. The transplant provides the patient with "new" marrow containing stem cells that will grow, divide, and mature into all the blood cell lines needed.

We became familiar with some of the people with children receiving cancer treatment. You could look at each other and everything was understood without saying anything. One of the families I met from New York still had to travel a ways to the hospital for treatment as their ten year old daughter was diagnosed with cancer in her knee. While we were receiving treatment, one day I saw the mother crying as she started talking to me. She cried "How can I give them permission to cut off my daughter's leg, she is only ten years old"? I asked her if that was the only choice she had and she said that they were not sure if they could save her daughters leg. They had another procedure that was when the leg is cut off; her foot could be attached backwards to her knee to help her with an artificial leg that would come later. She said she had worked in the operating room before and she could not stand for that to be done to her daughter. I really did not know what to say to this mother as I was really struggling myself with my own child's illness. I asked her to let me pray with her and to ask God to save her daughters leg. I held her hand as we prayed, I hugged her and she thanked me. I later saw her in the outpatient clinic with her daughter receiving chemotherapy. I saw that the daughter's leg was saved. We smiled together and she mentioned that she was told her daughter's leg would stay in remission for approximately ten years and the cancer would probably return. She was thankful for that because she said by then her daughter would be able to make her own decisions about her leg amputation. I rarely saw her because our schedules were not always the same. I saw a little boy that had the surgery with the foot attached to his knee. I tried not to stare but I thought it was amazing to have a foot put on backwards in order to assist with the fitting of an artificial limb. I also met a little girl that had an ambiblical cord transplant done. She told me that her donor was from Africa. A lot of the things you see at the Sloan Kettering Hospital were amazing to the eye and saddening at the same time. Some times what you see there would leave you with an impact that you can't ever forget.

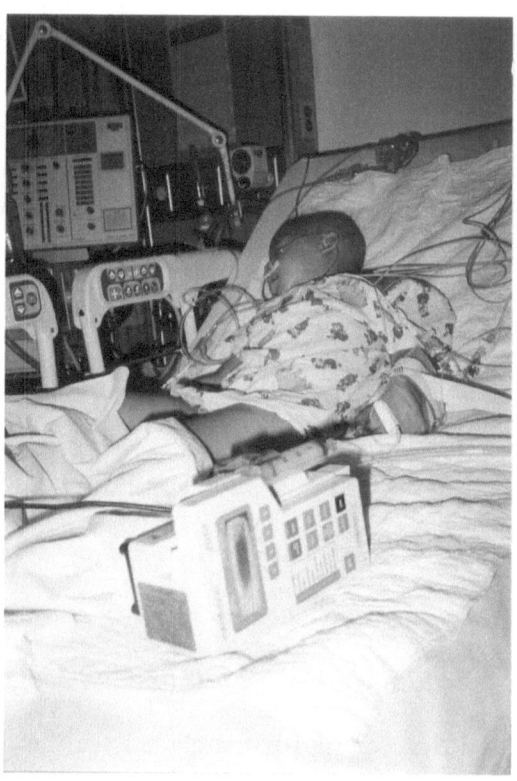

The Bone Marrow Transplant

Now that Asia has finished eight rounds of chemotherapy, it was time for her to start her bone marrow treatment. By this time she'd already been hospitalized approximately eleven times, not to include her numerous outpatient visits. To start her bone marrow treatment, Asia had to receive radioactive materials to kill any neuroblastoma cancer cells that may still exist after taking eight rounds of chemo, which killed her bone marrow, and was given back after being stored. We were told that if her body does not recover, she would die because this procedure would kill her entire immune system. For so many days the doctor would come in and insert a radioactive material into her central line in her chest. He'd come back later to check the radioactive levels. At this time we were not allowed to hold her and a shield was placed between us to help prevent us from being exposed to the radiation. Cafeteria workers would leave our food trays at the door because they weren't allowed in. Every time Asia had to receive treatment, I would go into prayer asking God to help

my child go through it. I went up to her bed to see how she was

doing on a regular basis. She knew I was not supposed to hug her

but she reached to hug me anyway. She understood why the doctor

told us that, so she responded well through it. She was real attached

to us. We stayed close to her, assuring her that she was not alone.

I assisted her when it was time for her to eat. She could not leave

the room until her radioactive levels went down. The doctor told

us that after about two days after she had received her radioactive

medication that if we could see her she would look like a light bulb

lit up due to the amount of radiation that she has inside of her. He

also told us not to hold her for long periods of time when we leave

and not to wash her clothes with ours. We were told that she would

most likely be returning to intensive care due to her immune system

being completely gone, and we could lose her if her blood counts

don't recover at this point. As the doctor would come in to check

Asia's radioactive levels, he was amazed how she sat up in her bed

as he stated "I am amazed at this kid". He asked us "what are you

doing for this kid"? He said usually by this point of treatment the

child is lying down not feeling well. I knew it was God. The doctor

said "whatever you are doing keep doing it". So many kids had

cardiac arrests when having these radioactive materials injected into

their bodies and their hospital stays were very long. Asia knew I was

praying for her as she would pay very close attention to me. I think
she was seeing how well we were taking care of her. I remember one
day I told Asia my back was hurting and she put her arms around my
neck and said "mama its going to be alright, I will pray for God to
heal you Amen". She was so considerate and concerned about people
that were helping her while she was also such a sensitive child. It was
like she could read me without me saying a word. I would try not to
cry in front of her because it bothered her to see me sad. I did not
want anything to affect her getting well, so when I cried I would do
it in another room or away from her. Asia said to me "mama do you
remember the day the pastor prayed for me"? I told her yes and she
said "it made me feel better". I knew Asia had noticed something
happened to her when she was prayed for. The doctor told us that
Asia's radioactive levels were really high and as soon as they come
down to a certain level that we'd be able to leave, but not until then
because her radiation level was too high to be exposed to others. We
were in the hospital December 6, 2000 thru December 13, 2000 and
were told we could be released to the Ronald McDonald House but
could not leave the state of New York due to her dangerous state.
We had to take her back to the outpatient clinic in about two days
to have her blood levels checked and to see what state her immune
system was in. We still had to keep her somewhat isolated. She then
developed a runny nose and this was dangerous with no immune

system. We carried her into the outpatient clinic to have her checked

and they immediately put her in a room by herself because she was

very susceptible to disease and germs. The doctor looked at her and

predicted that she probably had a respiratory infection and would

probably have to be hospitalized. They checked her mucus for

infection and the doctor realized that she didn't have a respiratory

infection. This was ironic because she had no immune mechanism

working at this time. He told us to return to the Ronald McDonald

House and keep her confined and away from people. Se we kept

her in our room until our return to the hospital in two days. If she

was to develop a fever we were to bring her back right away. The

doctors expected her to be admitted to intensive care, but thanks to

God her counts began to recover. Howbeit this kind goeth not out

but by prayer and fasting (Matthew 17:21). The doctors planned to

restore her bone marrow on December 28, 2000. While closely being

watched the outpatient visits continued.

Now after long waiting and constant outpatient visits the

time came to return her bone marrow back to her. It was infused

intravenously through her central line. It normally has garlic like

odor which is the smell of the drug used to protect the marrow

cells while they are frozen. After it was infused, she vomited, which

was expected to happen. Asia would once again have to be given neupogen injections to speed up the growth of her white blood cells

in the bone marrow. This procedure called for needles injected into

her little legs four to fifteen days. So much pain to endure for her

and the family. It really hurts to see your child walk around with

bruises from shots that you as a parent had to give in order to help

them survive. It was still December 2000, and we would have our

first Christmas in New York. We made arrangements for Chassity

to fly to New York in order for all of us to be together. I told them

we would have our own Christmas again when we get back home.

The Ronald McDonald House had many special things going on for

the kids and families on Christmas. They also arranged for Santa

Claus to come. The bill collectors were calling and the bills were

due but the most important thing to us was the lives of our children.

Our mortgage was behind and we were facing foreclosure. Dad

was borrowing money from friends, banks, relatives and also from

pawning. None of the organizations would continuously pay or

assist us with our mortgage. I went to apply for food stamps and

was rejected because our income was considered too high. If we

could receive any food stamps at all I was told it would be only about

ten dollars. I told the person at the Social Services building that a

situation like this should override the guidelines for food stamps

because it was a catastrophic situation. I said to the worker if this

would happen to you, how would you take care of your family? Even though he understood I still left with no assistance. I wrote some church organizations and received a gift card. I was told by some ministries that they did not help situations like this. I even sent them a letter from the doctor so they could check out my request for help, the answer was still no. When you walk a long journey you become alone because many people begin to drop off. The friends that you do have can only help but so much. We did not have any rich friends. I used credit cards for medications, airplane flights, and other necessities we couldn't afford. Our lives changed dramatically which also made our minds deranged. Can you imagine going home today and tomorrow having a totally different life? Just as I said in the beginning, you never think it will be you. We no longer had the regular every day continuous lives just going to work and watching our children have a normal life. We were robbing Peter to pay Paul and wondering how we could come up with money just to stay above water. It was no more staying on top of things. It was time to know that things would be worse by the day.

It was such a blessing for the Ronald McDonald House to have some meals but in between we had to buy our food and in Manhattan, New York and the cost of living there is very high. A one room apartment there is really small but costs about two thousand dollars a month. Trying to survive there was not easy.

After the bone marrow transplant, we had to wait for Asia's immune system to recover in order to leave New York. The stay went on for about six to eight weeks, until the doctor told us we could return to our home in Virginia. Now we were back at home returning twice a week to our local hospital for necessary platelets and blood checks. As Asia's bone marrow transplant now seemed to be doing ok, we had to return back to Sloan Kettering hospital again for monoclonal antibody treatments also known as (3F8). Monoclonal antibodies are tumor cells injected into a mouse to stimulate production of B cells, which produce different types of antitumor antibodies. Antibodies are used to help diagnose cancers hidden in the body. Radioactive substances are attached to monoclonal antibodies that recognize and target cancer cells. The antibodies are injected into the body to find cancer cells to bind to them. When 3F8 is injected into a patient's blood stream, it travels and attaches to the neuroblastoma cells. The attachment of 3F8 to a neuroblastoma cell serves as a signal to patients own immune system to attack and kill the neuroblastoma. The side effects of the antibody are severe pain, skin rash, fever, and high or low blood pressure. Due to the radiation, there is potential damage to vital organs of the body.

Another Treatment: The Antibody

Once again it was time to book our flights and change out our clothes that were already in the suitcase from the last trip. Our luggage stayed packed and placed by the font door. As you had to stay prepared to go to the hospital at any given time. Airplane flights occurred every two weeks for this type of treatment. The airport itself was another stressful experience. I had to make sure I had Asia's medications on board. As we were riding on the plane I looked over at Asia and she had a set of headphones on listening to some music. She had an expression on her face which showed curiosity as to what am I going to go through this time, but as I said she never once complained. We were on our way back for this treatment and Asia was given premedication for pain before given the antibody. The antibody was given intravenously through her central line through an IV drip which took about thirty minutes. She needed to be there approximately three hours when the 3F8 attaches to a nerve cell, a message is sent to the brain and pain begins toward the middle or the end, and more pain medication is given such as dilaudid, morphine. Benadryl is given for itching and rash because she began to cry and scream how bad it hurts. We stood there totally helpless. The pain can continue for hours after the treatment. The pain medication helped but some days the level of pain was so high they'd already given her the maximum that she could take. She received antibodies for two weeks and then we would return back home again. This was to continue until she'd developed a HAMA, human anti-mouse antibodies. She would say "mama, start praying and she would reach to hold my hand, crying about the pain she was in. She would like her stomach rubbed also. It was so hard to go through, seeing her as well as other children crying that were going through the same treatment. When we would leave after the treatments, she'd be emotionally disturbed, very irritable and in pain from all the medications that were given to her. It would take about two hours for her to calm down and be herself again. She would cry all the way from the hospital to the Ronald McDonald House. It seemed nothing would please her until she calmed down. It would take us time to unwind ourselves after going through these days of treatment, because it brought on great amounts of stress as well as loss of appetites and sleep. Sometimes the stress would be so heavy that it was hard to pray because praying consisted of taking about the pain which brought on more pressure. As I felt the pressure against

my head, I would say Lord you already know what I am trying to
say but just talking to you it hurts so badly and the more I say the
more the pressure builds up. Sometimes you can't even say a word.
We traveled to New York for about nine more additional months
for antibody treatments. Asia then developed a HAMA. In between
these trips to New York and returning home, she was to be taken to
our local hospital for labs again, checking her blood levels, platelets
and to see if she still had her HAMA. Once the HAMA is developed
the 3F8 treatments are stopped. However the HAMA can disappear
and 3F8 treatments will resume. HAMA is a good sign that the
patient has developed an immune response against neuroblastoma
which is a good thing. Although some kids relapse during 3F8
treatment. Most patients who have received chemotherapy for short
time before 3F8 treatment do not make HAMA because the immune
system is too weak. Some children never develop Hama's and
antibody treatment continues on for two years.

Every three months from the date of diagnosis Asia is tested with
cat scans, bone scans and bone marrow aspirations checking to see
the status of the cancer, because even though she was in remission, we
were told Neuroblastoma is known to come back. Every time Asia
went through these tests, she could not eat, infact none of us ate until
she could eat. That was to help her out. If the test was scheduled

for late in the day that was too hard for Asia to deal with so we tried
to arrange her test early. We started flying to Sloan Kettering for her
test because they were done much faster and efficient than our local
hospital. The Children's Hospital of Kings Daughter in Virginia
would request Asia drink eight ounces of liquid that was required
for a cat scan and Sloan Kettering had a drink for the same test that
required only half a cup. That was wonderful because it is very hard
to get a small child to consume some of the things the hospital may
require for a child. Also when she had MRI's she had to be put
under anesthesia, which required being inside a machine for forty five
minutes to an hour for the completion of the test that's really long for
a small child which feels scared inside a machine all by themselves.
Some adults cannot take MRI due to claustrophobia. We tried to
help Asia with the less suffering as possible; she was already going
through so much. Her life was living in and out of the hospital. The
chemotherapy caused Asia to have some tooth decay and had to have
several teeth extracted, at the same time the dentist told us her teeth
had developed beyond her age. Chemotherapy leaves side effects
even after taking it. Her trip to her local dentist was horrible. She
continued to say that her mouth was in pain, but the dentist said
it was only because she was scared. We explained to him that Asia
required more pain medication than the average patient her size but
it seems that was ignored. We later took our other child Chassity to

the same dentist and she said she felt pain the whole time although he

was supposed to have numbed her mouth. After having two children

complain of the same thing we knew they were telling the truth

so se decided to have Asia's dental work done at Sloan Kettering.

They seemed to know what to do for children with cancer and were

familiar with the problems. They would arrange her tooth extractions

during one of her procedures while she was under anesthesia. As

for Chassity we found her another dentist. It was so much more

convenient to have Asia's mouth done in New York since she was

there so often.

Now that Asia has her HAMA, her antibody treatment was

finished and we were hoping she stayed in remission. We would

still have to constantly have her blood levels checked of see if she

still had her HAMA as well as her platelet counts and blood levels.

Before we left Sloan Kettering we asked if Asia could have her central

line removed from her chest and they said yes. When we told Asia

that her line could be removed the smile on her face was worth a

million dollars. She had to be put under anesthesia to have her line

removed. Now there would be no more dressing changes and she

could get to play in the swimming pool and try to experience what

it feels like to be a normal child. Asia had kept her original lines the

whole time because we were fortunate that they never got infected, if they did they would have required replacements under anesthesia. Some children had multiple lines put in due to infection. Since she no longer had central lines, she had her blood drawings from her arms, which was another painful situation to watch because she still had to have frequent blood drawings. She would cry every time. Her little arms would bruise from the needles. I would put Emla cream on her arm before arriving at the clinic to help with the pain of the needle. Asia was then put on an Acutance, a medication that consisted of 60mg gel caps. She was prescribed to take three capsules in the morning and three in the evening. She was so young and did not swallow pills; this was a very difficult task so I would try to put them in food such as Jell-O or pudding. I had to then burst the caps and squeeze the liquid into something to help her swallow them. She hated them; she'd tell me how nasty it was. Dad and I tasted it and she was definitely right. The gel inside the cap would come through anything you added it with. We continued to give it to her; it made everybody a nervous wreck trying to get this medication inside her little body. She was to take for fourteen days and then she could have a two week break from it. Her calcium and liver functions had to be checked due to the side effects of this medication. She hated to see you coming with the medicine and would sometimes gag and could not swallow it. This medication is known to help with cancer. One of Accutane's greatest side effects is very dry skin and chapped lips.

We had to use oatmeal bath products and plenty of moisturizers to help with her skin. Her skin became very sensitive.

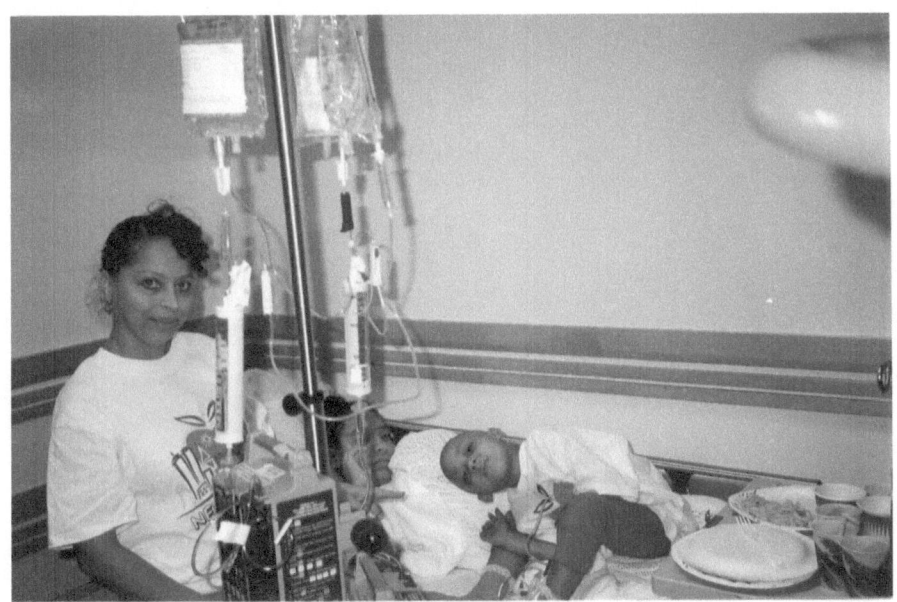

Asia Enrolls into School

When Asia turned four she wanted to go to school. This was like a miracle for all of us to see her this way. We enrolled her into pre-school. She wanted to experience riding the school bus. What a smile she had on her face when she was to carry a back pack and go to school as so many kids take it for granted. She was a great example of someone who just truly appreciated life. Dad took pictures of her first day. You could see how proud she was to be able to do this. She felt she had achieved a big accomplishment because most children with her illness never got to see the inside of a school. She handled her first day of school so well. She was taken to school at first because this school did not have a school bus pick up in our areas. When I went to leave her, she looked at me like she did not want me to leave her, but still made it though it. She was transferred to another school that did have school bus pick up. She would get on the bus and look out the window until the bus drove off. She would be so happy when the bus dropped her off, as we were standing there waiting to greet her. She really appreciated life in such a wonderful way. After a while she wanted Dad to start carrying her back to school. She looked forward to him being there. It was good to see Asia outside riding in her Barbie Jeep and being able to play like everyone else.

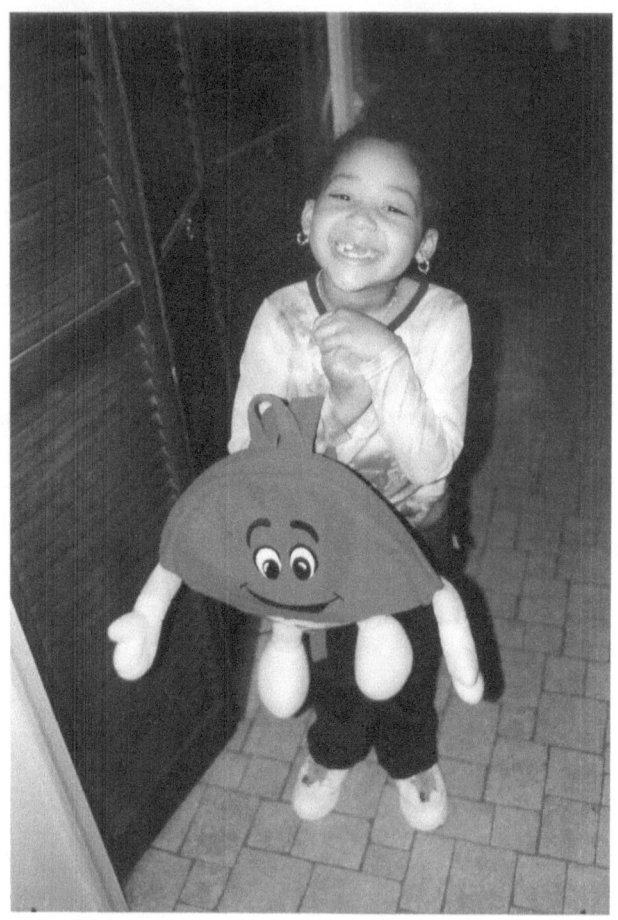

The Petting Zoo

One day after dad picked Asia up from school, they went to the SPCA (petting zoo) to look at the dogs, cats, alligators, ostriches, chickens, llama, leopards, lions and jaguar cats. Of course some of them were caged but Asia was an animal lover. She went fishing one day with dad and after dad caught the fish she told him to put it back in the water to let it live. Asia wanted a kitten and while visiting there, she spotted one that she liked. She showed her father the one she wanted. He told her that they would go home and bring mom back to see it. He said she cried as they came home because she has set her heart on that kitten. Then they came home and she told me all about it she was ready to go back to the petting zoo. When we went back, she headed straight for the cage that the cat was in. She didn't need to look any further because her mind was made up. She wanted to take him home, but I told her we still had to think about it. When we got home she began to cry, she knew if someone else went there that they may take him home and she would lose him.

Her dad had spoken to one of the workers at the SPCA and told her

that Asia was interested in that cat, and stated he'd return tomorrow.

I thought later that if someone else gets that kitten it would be hard

for me to live with myself should something happen to Asia and

she not have her heart's desire. The next day she remembered that

we were suppose to take her back to the petting zoo. I told her we

would stop by there on the way back from her doctor's visit. She fell

asleep in the car, but we stopped as promised, and her father stayed

in the car while I went to purchase the kitten. It was like he was put

there for her, because the day before, he came right to her and stuck

his paw out of the cage continuously to touch her. It was as if they

had a connection. When I went in, I told the lady I was there to get

him. As she put him in a carrying box, he constantly stuck his paws

through the holes and his little eyes to look out. I put the box in the

back of the car as Asia was sleep. She awakened shortly to notice the

box was in the car. What a smile she had. When she let him out of

the box, he walked around as if he had already been living with us.

He was a calm, compassionate, tabby cat that was only three months

old. He was so loveable. Asia named him Oliver from the movie

Oliver & Company. It was the cat she had already described that she

wished for. She always wanted a cat that would lye on her bed and be

very gentle. He was all that she had ordered. He was very smart as

when the alarm clock went off in the morning he would use his paw to touch you to wake you up and during the night he would come and check on you. You could hear his little motor running which would sometimes wake you up. He would come in with a sound announcing his presence when he entered the room. It was like he was made for her. Of course, Chassity being an animal lover as well adored him and was his caretaker also. Oliver became suddenly sick and died December 2005. I thought it was strange as cats usually live a long time but Oliver only lived three years. My husband says Asia came to get him for her Christmas present, as he left six days before Christmas. Chassity and Asia also had Susie, the family dog, who is a great protector of the house and has moved everywhere we've been.

Asia's Wish, Almost Ruined

Now that Asia is in remission, we thought it would be a good time for her to receive her wish from the "Make a Wish Foundation" which is an organization that pays for every child with a lift threatening illness to live a wish they'd like to come true. The wish was totally up to her, they send a representative out to talk with the child and ask them what they would like to do. Asia said she wanted to go to Disney World. The representative told her he would set up her trip and get back with her. He later gave her a calendar to put a sticker on everyday as her date became closer. She was so excited. I told her it was because of her that we would all get to go to Disney world and I thanked her letting her know she was a very special person. Asia has been in remission for almost a year, though treatment steadily continued. As we were preparing for Florida, Asia still had to be seen regularly at our local Children's Hospital clinic for constant lab work. This disease had to be closely monitored. She begin to complain that one of her arms were hurting. We carried her to the doctor and informed him that she

had been complaining of arm pain. During the doctor's visit, he

told us that she needed to be biopsied, which consisted of the use

of a needle under anesthesia in order to take a sample of the tissue

in the arm to see if the Neuroblastoma was back. This of course

felt like I was being stabbed again. We're all feeling as though the

bottom of our lives was dropping again. After all the treatment and

pain that she had already been through, we thought this couldn't be

happening. The test came back positive for Neuroblastoma. The

doctor recommended radiation to the arm which would give her pain

relief. We proceeded with the radiation and this time and received

the radiation in Virginia. It turned her arm dark as if she had been

burned, so we decided in the future if she needed further radiation

we would have it done at the hospital in New York. The doctor

needed to mark her arm for radiation explained to us that she would

have to be put under anesthesia everyday, radiation would be at least

three weeks. We explained to the doctor that she had already had

radiation before, so anesthesia would not be necessary. Due to her

being so young, he stated she would not keep still. We proceeded to

assure him she does not need to be put to sleep. Not at all convinced

the doctor accepted our proposal. The doctor was very surprised

because it was performed with no anesthesia. Like I said earlier, she

was an older woman in a young body. The radiation stopped the

pain and and she began to use her arm again. I thought this was just
too much for anybody to go through. After radiation, we decided it
was time for a trip to New York to see what the doctor's there had to
say about the Neuroblastoma coming back. The doctor, of course
proceeded with further testing, bone marrow aspiration, bone scan,
cat san and blood tests. The test confirmed that the Neuroblastoma
was back. The doctor had an angry look on his face; he too was
disappointed as well as us. It hurts to see a child fight so hard only
to have the bomb drop again. The doctor stated that Neuroblastoma
would be more aggressive and of course she would have to do more
chemotherapy treatments and another bone marrow transplant. Asia
had enough bone marrow stored to do two more transplants which
was unusual. Because she had already had so many harsh chemicals
already put in her body her immune system would be affected even
more upon responding. Relapsed disease was worst, due to the cancer
recognizing the chemotherapies she had already had. This tore our
lives into shreds again as we were so looking forward to Asia beating
this disease. I wanted to cry but couldn't in front of her. This news
was once again very devastating to hear. We explained to the doctor
that Asia was scheduled to go to Disney World, he said it would be a
good idea for her to go on her trip before we started treatment, since
she had no central line in her chest. That too would be inserted in
order to start treatment again. We decided to go on to Disney world

and let Asia have all the fun she could have, feeling free as a bird without any treatment intervening. Asia was so excited about her trip. She had something to look forward to after all she had gone through.

Our airplane flight was scheduled at four o'clock in the morning; the limousine would arrive between three o'clock to pick us up for Asia's trip. It was so early in the morning. She looked like she was still sleepy, but she was very aware that she was on her way to her planned trip. As we were riding in the limousine, we took pictures of Asia and Chassity sitting in the limousine. When we arrived at the airport, after an hour ride, a sponsor from the Make a Wish Foundation met us there and stayed with us until it was time for us to get on the airplane. By this time Asia was wide awake. When we arrived to Florida and as Asia were entering the Airport, there were people waiting for her with a giant greeting card welcoming her. Wow, did that make her feel special. They told Asia where she would be staying and escorted us to our rental car which we drove to the Give Kids the World Village. We were told not to worry about putting the gas back in the car. Asia was so alive. I could see and feel her excitement. It made my heart smile to see my child who's gone through so much finally have some happy moments. It would bring tears to your eyes. As we were finding our way to the village, we enjoyed the beautiful weather, palm trees, and seeing oranges hanging

off the trees. It was February 2001 and it was cold in Virginia. We

arrived in Florida with coats on. People knew right away that we had

come from somewhere where it was cold. We were greeted with a

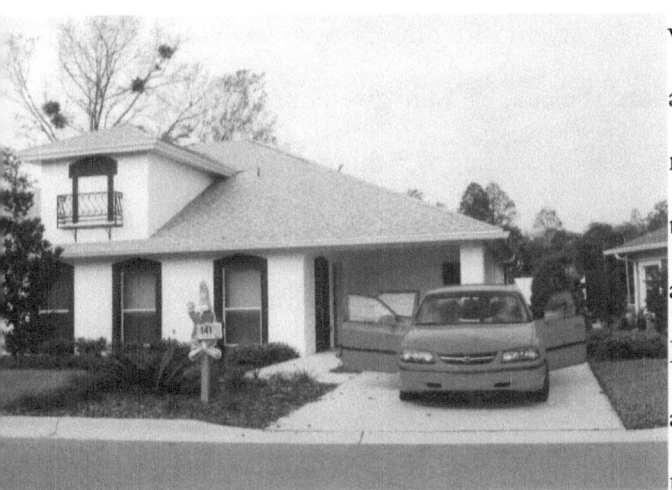

very pleasant invitation
at the village. They
really welcomed us as
they presented Asia
and Chassity with a
Disney World stuffed
animal character and
told me to put my purse
away, because it wasn't

needed there. I thought wow this is extremely nice. This is really

living. I mean how many places you can go without using your purse

(monies). They proceeded to escort us through the village. I was

surprised because our stay area was just like a private condominium

rather than a hotel room. We had our own kitchen with food already

in the refrigerator, two bedrooms, and televisions in every room, two

bathrooms and a dining area. Every day someone would come to the

room to leave a toy for Asia and Chassity. The village consisted of

a movie theatre with all the popcorn and drinks that you could eat,

three swimming pools, a place to eat in the morning and dinner in the evening. Another eating place had hot dogs and drinks all day, an

ice cream parlor and train rides for the kids. It was so nice just being

there. The village was set up for kids with life threatening illnesses. I

was told that a man that had a sick child decided to set the village up

for children with illnesses. As we got into our room we were told all

the rules, in order to get into the gate we were given our passwords

and this was for security as well. Another nice thing about it was how

some of the people that worked there too also had disabilities, so they

could really relate to the children. They were all so compassionate

and it seemed they really understood the difficult lives the children

were experiencing.

We were so tired by
the time we arrive the first
day we decided to head
out to Disney World the
next morning. The tickets
for the parks were also
given to us as we arrived
at the village. It was so
heavenly to have our own
private place, nice inside
and out. Before we left for
the Disney parks, we went

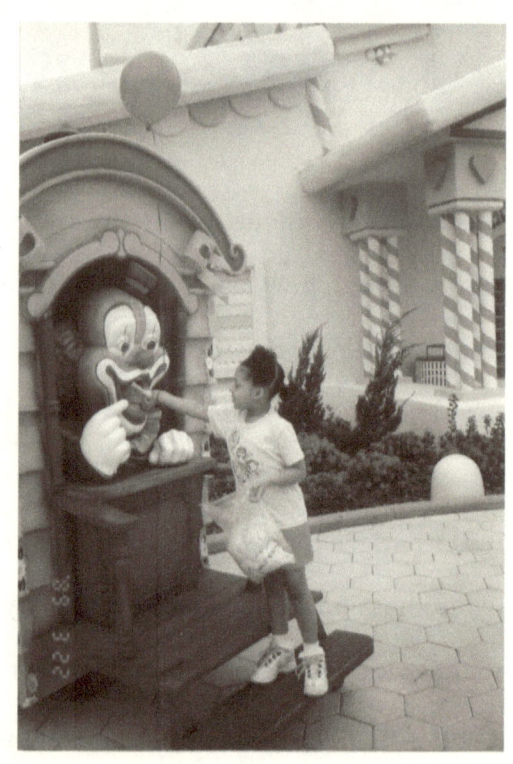

to have our breakfast at the food kitchen. It was set up like a buffet, plenty to eat, and the people were so friendly. All of us set there with such excitement as we had went through so much to get to this point and wondered at times if Asia would get her wish. Asia was so happy as well as Chassity. We took so many pictures. We were also given a video camera as well to video our trip. The Kids Village transferred it to a tape for us. It felt like a dream had come true. While we could finally focus on Asia's happiness as oppose to what we knew we had to look forward to. Asia was so anxious and energetic. She had plans for us everyday. Asia fell in love with the talking trash can at the Kids Village. It had a clown face and when you put trash in it, the clown would say how good the food was and to please give me more. Asia really enjoyed putting the trash in. After eating, we all got into the car, which by the way was brand new. Asia was given a button by the village to wear while at the Disney World Park which gave her the privileges of not having to wait in line for any rides. This benefit was because the kids could not wait for long periods of times due to their illnesses. Asia did some walking but we still had to use the stroller. We went to Universal Studios for two days which was her favorite, along with Sea World, Magical Kingdom and two other Parks. Asia also had a personal visit with the Disney characters, Mickey and Minnie, Cinderella, Goofy, Snow White and the seven dwarfs and many others as she was escorted to them and had personal

pictures done as well. She attended Merlin the magician show and
was chosen to pull the sword out and was given a special ribbon. We
also got to watch the Little Mermaid show and
visit Nickelodeon along with Blue Clue's. We
then saw a live Nickelodeon show in which
Asia and Chassity got to sit in on. Another one
of Asia favorite was ET, which we rode several
times. Everything seemed so magical. Believe it
or not Asia liked the roller coaster and also rode
it many times as well. After a long day at the
Disney Park we were very tired upon our return
to the village. We decided to eat at the park,
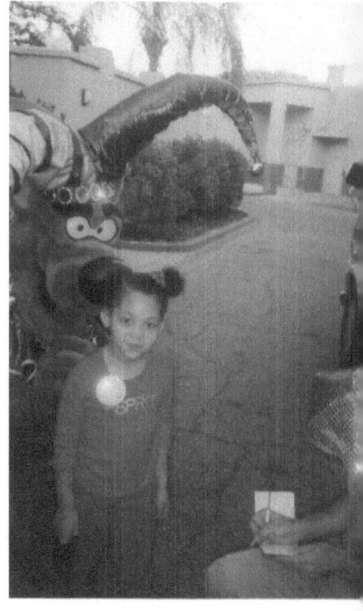
having so much fun, we lost track of dinner time at the village. The
next morning it was breakfast time again and we stuffed ourselves
to leave for the Disney Park again. Today we would visit a different
park to return earlier for our buffet dinner at the village. The food
was so good, and of course, we could get ice cream until nine o'clock
at night. Asia also had a date with the kids village rabbit (Mayor
Clayton) which comes and tucks you into bed. She was extremely
excited about that as she prepared herself for it. He also tucked
Chassity in as well. It was just so relaxing not to have to cook or
clean for a week. We went to the parks at Disney up until it was time
to come back home. We began to pack the night before and the next

morning after breakfast, Asia refused to get into the car and told us that she wanted to move there. We said well what do we do about your grandmother that we left behind, she replied, "she can move with us here". She cried as her trip was coming to an end, but we finally talked her into getting into the car by ultrally picking her up and trying to explain to her that we had to go home so that we could fly to New York for her appointment to see her doctor. We then returned the rental car and caught our flight back to Virginia.

Back to Reality: Treatments Start Again

We arrived home waiting for our next adventure, which was our doctor visit. As the doctor had told us before, Asia had to start chemotherapy again and would have another central line put in her chest. The sail on our boats were really down. Flying back to New York to Sloan Kettering Hospital meant a long stay. Asia began her chemotherapy and another bone marrow transplant to follow. It was like life was taken away from us again and each time the doctor would say we could loose her. It was so scary and painful to experience this process again. We knew her immune system had already been damaged from the previous chemotherapies and radiation treatments. Asia's chemotherapy treatment this time was different; she was given chemotherapy for so many days and then given her new bone marrow. The chemotherapies were changed due to the cancer being smart enough to recognize the previous chemotherapy. Of course she lost her hair again and her immune system dropped. It was the start of another long journey. During our stays in the hospital with Asia at

Sloan Kettering we were delivered two food trays for breakfast, lunch

and dinner. One was for the parent and one for the patient. Even

during our outpatient visits we were served lunch everyday and had

access to coffee, juices, cereal and milk, some fruit and tea as well. I

must say they really look out for the families and understand very well

the financial state this illness put on them. They realize the families

really need a helping hand. We are so grateful that they served as part

of our survival.

While receiving chemotherapy or blood platelets as an outpatient,

there was always entertainment for the kids to occupy them. There

were clowns and recreational activities. In some instances the play

room allowed you to roll your IV pole along with you. They had

many gifts for the children. People would come to the child's bedside

to give your child something to play with during treatment. They'd

also play with them if the child was ok with it. It made the children

feel like it wasn't just a hospital. During holidays there were always

parties for the kids as well. Characters walk around and entertained

as some people would play instruments and sing to them. There were

also colored televisions at each child's bed for them to watch.

While Asia was receiving treatment, a nurse asked Asia if she

would like to have Kimberly Williams visit her. She played in

Help! My Child Has Cancer

the movie "Father of the Bride". Asia said yes. She came in the
room, talked with Asia and took a picture with her. I thought how
wonderful for her to take time out of her life to visit kids that were
fighting for their lives. I knew Asia was special, I would see her get to
do things despite her illness that other kids would never experience.
But what a price to pay. During our travels to New York we met
another angel; Gabriel that worked in a health store that helped us
as he took an interest in Asia's illness. He had also experienced some
type of cancer and understood her life and what it was like. He was
very helpful and thoughtful. I thought it was amazing how he did
not know us but it was as if we already knew each other and were
family. God does work in mysterious ways.

While waiting for Asia's blood, more shots were given to her
to help her white blood cells recover, in order to help her immune
system. It took even longer this time and the hospital stay was much
longer. The hospital stay was getting to all of us as Asia began to
get very agitated. Dad and I began to feel the prison life. We felt
as though we were at our limits and told the doctor that we had an
urge to leave and would take Asia. He asked us to please stay and
wait it out as it would be better for Asia. I was beginning to feel
claustrophobic; I could only imagine how Asia felt. We were told
that her counts could possibly not return, which made it hard on

us. We wondered why we are losing our child this time. We waited longer and her counts began to come back, but they had to be a certain number for her to leave the hospital. When they finally came up, we were told we could return to the Ronald McDonald House, but we still had to make constant visits back to the outpatient clinic for blood transfusions and platelets. We would not know if the bone marrow was a success until she completely recovered. She had to take special medications because of the bone marrow transplant, so we could not leave New York anytime, since the home hospital did not handle bone marrow transplants. Once Asia recovered we went home only to return in about six weeks for a bone scan, bone marrow aspiration, MRI and cat scans to see if she was again in remission. We finally got home for a short visit again.

We wondered what the outcome was for us as we went back to New York for testing. We were told she was still showing some Neuroblastoma cells, we just wanted to disappear from the face of the earth after hearing this news. Now the doctor recommended oral chemotherapy (Etoposide) by mouth to keep the cancer cells from spreading. The oral chemotherapy took some of her hair out after it growed back in some places it thinned. She took the chemotherapy for a little while but began to develop pain. The doctor in New York then recommended she start IV chemotherapy (Irrinotecan) as an outpatient at our local hospital which would help with the pain. While we were in New York we also sought out another doctor at Meridian Medical which treated cancer, but used some different medications that were non toxic. It's believed to be active against cancer by reprogramming aberrantly programmed cancer cells to become normal cells again. The doctor wished we had gotten to him sooner as her state of cancer had really progressed. The medication that was prescribed for her was not covered by any insurance companies; therefore we had to pay out of pocket. The medicine had to be ordered from a special pharmaceutical company. The doctor also recommended shark cartilage and had to be shipped on ice in small glass bottles. The shark cartilage and tributyrate was about three hundred dollars each and since we had no pay checks coming in credit cards was all we had to buy this medicine.

On our way back home with these medications we returned home to start IV Irrinotecan chemotherapy twice a week and in between there were visits for blood counts, platelets and transfusions as the chemotherapy was taking its effects. We discussed going to the Meridian Medical with our other doctors at Sloan Kettering before going. Trying to get Asia to take the medications was a tough fight as Asia did not swallow pills and she had to take five 500mg of tributyrate three times a day. I had to mix it with foods, juices or anything I thought would help her swallow the medication. She would gag when she tried to take it. It thought if she would just try it but we only got through a half of the bottle and she started refusing to take it completely as the gagging reflex increased even more. I tasted the medication and it did have a real horrible taste, and of course it did not come in a liquid. As a result we then went along with the IV Irrinotecan. The Irrinotecan side effects were diarrhea which was to the point that I had to apply Vaseline to her rectum again to help with the irritation and soreness. I cannot say if the Tributyrate helped because Asia never finished the whole bottle, and the state of her cancer had already significantly progressed. I thought if I could get her to try it maybe things would turn around. Being very desperate to save my child's life we were still looking for options to save our daughter's life, we called a hospital in Israel, which was not very successful, as we were stuck in New York in September 2001, the day the World Trade Center was hit by an airplane and every telephone call was monitored. We called the hospital but because of the disaster we couldn't go because all airports, buses, trains and taxicabs were all stopped. It was strange to be able to count the people on the streets of New York as it is always hard to walk without touching someone. We too had received our 911 because this time the doctor told us that Asia was leaving us. I felt we really received our 911 in January 1999 when Asia was first diagnosed. At least we were stuck close to the hospital and could walk there because people that had to come from Brooklyn, Queens, etc could not get into Manhattan due to the disaster that was going on. They had to use the closest hospital to them or not receive their treatment, the blood supply was limited and children with cancer needed many transfusions. The treatment in Israel was not a definite cure but we were trying to do everything we could to save Asia. Months later, though we were taking the Irrinotecan, she began to complain of pain again. Irrinotecan was said to slow the cancer cells down but would not put her into remission. Now at this time Tylenol 3 pain medication was added along with the Irrinotecan to help with pain. We began again to search for other treatments to help with this horrible disease. As we were discussing treatments with our local doctor he spoke with us about a treatment named (MIBG) Meta-Iodo-benzyl-Guanidine, a form of iodine that is radioactive, killing cancer cells by the radioactivity. We then talked with the doctors in New York as well because this treatment wasn't performed there nor Virginia. This treatment was practiced in Philadelphia Children's Hospital. We decided to check into the treatment still trying hard to keep Asia alive. The doctors from New York spoke with the doctor in Philadelphia as well as our local doctor and a scheduled appointment was set up. Before leaving to go to the hospital in Philadelphia the local physician stated that he would need a bone marrow aspiration

done in order for the new physician to see how her cells were doing. We had the bone marrow aspiration done and prepared our luggage and drove her to the Philadelphia Children's Hospital to see if this type of treatment would be of any help to her.

A Day in Philadelphia

We met with the physician to discuss the procedure. He
explained that she would be given the MIBG intravenously, which
would be injected into the body slowly. It would take about one hour
and hospitalization would be required for a few days. She would have
a special suite to herself but they only wanted one parent in the room
due to the high exposure of radiation. He went on to explain that
most of the iodine is taken up by the cancer cells but that her good
cells would be affected as well and the rest of the iodine passes out
through the urine. He also said she would not be able to be released
until a certain amount of radioactivity in her body was reduced to
a specific level. It kind of reminded me of her first bone marrow
transplant. There was a television and bathroom in the suite but
she would not be able to come out after the treatment, she'd need to
avoid the public or close interaction with us because of the radiation.
It was safe for a parent to be in the room with them but not to hold
or sit with her for long periods of time. Sleeping beside the child

during treatment was not recommending either. Some children of older ages may be able to stay alone but small children usually did not want to, especially Asia. No assistance, no treatment was Asia's rule. This treatment is not done at many places so; of course there was a waiting list. They could only assist one child in a room at time. An opening was available as someone had cancelled for whatever reason. We sought to look into it. After explaining the procedure to us, we asked what would be the chances of her survival. He told us he needed to look at her bone marrow test. After examining it, he told us that her bone marrow had more cancer cells than normal cells and he did not understand how she was still here and walking around. He went on to say that Asia may not make it through the treatment because she did not have many good cells left that would be needed to survive, because the treatment would kill the small amount of good cells that she had left. This procedure also required a bone marrow rescue as Asia had one more left at the hospital in New York. The doctor also said after reviewing her bone marrow test, he couldn't understand why our doctor sent us there. We were so out done and we were just looking at her and thinking how could this be true? How could she be standing here talking and playing and have so little good cells in her body? I could not tell her that but our hearts were so torn and I wanted to cry so bad but couldn't because I could not let her see the hurt that I was carrying. Once again I asked myself "how could this be happening to us"? I remember her sitting

down with the doctor as he was talking to her and doing her check up

examination. He looked at her with such amazement but also told us

the he could not put her through it because she may not come back.

He said she had already been though so much and he wanted to just

let her live the rest of her days as happy as she could. Taking her

through this procedure could be our last days with her. I thought to

myself I could not live with the fact that I put her through that if and

she leaves us. Dad felt the same way. Dad was in despair as well but

was not showing it to Asia. As we would look at each other we could

both feel the same pain. One of the hardest parts of going through

this with Asia was the fact that she was so little and could not make

her own decisions, we as parents knew everything we decided upon,

had to live with it.

Looking For Answers

Asia and I was watching a movie one day about a woman that had cancer. As we were watching, I asked Asia if she was the woman would she want them to recessitate her or just leave her alone. Her reply was "mama whatever you have to do to keep me alive". I then knew Asia wanted to live but I also had my answer from her upon what she would like for me to do should this happen to her. After our meeting with the doctor we decided to come back home and not go through with the MIBG treatment. I thought maybe this treatment would have been helpful if she had it done at an earlier stage of her cancer. Some children did have the procedure and it helped but they were not cured. It sometimes had to be done more than one time. We were still seeking other treatments and still looking for a miracle as we could not accept our child was leaving us. I even called St Jude's Hospital and spoke with a physician to see if they had anything different to offer for Neuroblastoma cancer but they had nothing different and also did not do antibody treatment. I contacted them in the earlier state of her cancer. I surfed the internet

seeking all types of hospitals and treatments that were available for

Neuroblastoma.

Asia's pain began to become more frequent. She stopped walking

as much and would lie down a lot more. I continued giving her

Tylenol 3 more frequently. She began to feel extremely bad and

stopped walking altogether. She was lying in bed more so I knew

something was wrong. She felt so bad that she didn't want to be

moved around either so I knew the pain had escalated. I could

hardly bear to see this. I was feeling so desperate for help for her.

I met many other families during these hospital visits and travels

that also had children with Neuroblastoma. Two of the families we

bonded with also lived in Virginia. We could really relate as we were

going through the same thing. One of my local friends called me,

as we would call each other in between our hospital visits, to discuss

treatments and we shared advice. She happened to come home from

New York from carrying her child there only to get some things and

I told her Asia was not doing well at all. She told me to come on and

catch a ride with her and take Asia back to the New York Hospital. I

told my husband that this would be the best thing to do. Since Asia

did not feel like being moved around she would not be able to sit on a

plane ride at this state. Dad put her in the back seat, her lying down

and I in the back to continue the administration of pain meds as Dad
sat in the front. We had to pack very quickly. In order to get Asia
in the car we had to carry her on pillows. My friend liked driving
at night due to traffic, so we rode all night. I had to give her pain
meds every three hours to keep her comfortable as possible as she was
showing signs that she needed something stronger. When we arrived
it was daylight but I had to wait until she took more pain medication
in order to move her from the car to the stroller to carry her from
the Ronald McDonald House to the hospital. When we arrived
they saw the discomfort and pain that she was in and immediately
started giving her dosages of morphine through her central line and
she began to vomit because morphine will cause nausea. As she was
vomiting the nurses continued to tell her it was ok. In about an hour
Asia began to feel better. They continued to work with her pain until
the pain was gone. It was so good to see that somebody knew what to
do as my child was really suffering. After being watched we left and
strolled her back to the Ronald McDonald House. This time Asia
was put on a pain patch named Fentanyl. The patches cost about one
hundred eleven dollars a box, containing five patches to a box. One
to two was to be applied every seventy two hours. She was also given
pain medication to take by mouth for break through pain. Now
that her pain was under control we were returning home to our local
hospital and Asia would be continuing IV Irrinotecan.

Asia's Birthday

While sitting at home one evening after coming home from the hospital, we were watching television, Asia sitting in my lap, looked up at me and said "Mama I want to go home". I explained to her that we were at home, but she did not say anything else. Dad told me that one day they were playing with her horses and she stopped in the middle of their playing and told him she wanted to go home and then left the room. As he called her back to talk about what she had said once again the conversation was over. Asia's birthday was approaching and we brought her birthday presents. I tried to surprise her but when I returned with the gifts from the store (she was at home with Dad) she began to cry. I asked her why was she crying but she did not answer me. I wondered if she knew it was her last birthday. I think Asia was smart enough to realize time was the most precious gift, and the presents weren't, because she told me later that she wanted to go with me. It seemed she knew so much more than we did.

Now that we were back home, Chassity had a school program that she needed to attend. Chassity, Asia and I were all in the car on our way to drop Chassity off for her program, as Asia, and I were returning home. While sitting at a traffic light a Ford Explorer hits us in the back. Another car hits him the Ford Explorer putting us in a three car collision, I worried about whether Asia was hurt since she was sitting in the back seat. I wouldn't have been able to handle if I was to open the back door and she was hurt. I jumped out the car and opened the back door to see if she was alright. She had fallen asleep and did not even know we had been hit. I called out her name "Asia is you alright"? She said what happened? I told her we were involved in a car accident. A lady came to my car to see if we were alright saying "lady you must have had some serious angels around your car as you both should be dead". My car was a total loss and the driver that caused the car accident had no car insurance. So now my transportation was gone and the back of my trunk was smashed all the way to the back seat where Asia was lying. My plate was already full and now this.

Asia's Trip to the North Pole

Once again Asia was receiving chemotherapy and we were going
to our local hospital two to three times a week, in between those days
we were there for blood checks for platelets and blood transfusions. It
was Christmas time of December 2001 and Asia was invited to take
a trip to the North Pole in which, an airplane was to fly Asia and us
and other families around in the sky telling them they were on their
way to the North Pole to see Santa Claus, after an hour we landed
back at the airport and Santa was sitting there with bags of toys for
all of the kids. Asia and all the kids really had a good time, and the
smiles on their faces were worth it all. While it was time for Asia and
Chassity's Christmas at home, one of Asia's gifts from her dad was
her own piano/organ that already had songs programmed in it. She
was really happy about that gift. While we were exploring a lot of
the music and songs that were programmed, she fell in love with the
beauty and the beast song. While I was listening to it, I said to her "I
will always think of you every time I hear the song"; she just looked

at me with such a straight face and never said a word. She walked around and looked at all her new items. Asia was the beauty and the neuroblastoma was the beast.

The Irrinotecan Treatment

The Irrinotecan helped for a little while until Asia began to develop pain again. Before receiving the Irrinotecan, she had to receive pain medication IV because she would complain when we arrived at the clinic. The nurse gave her some pain medication but Asia still complained. The local doctor told us the pain was a sign of the disease progressing. As Asia was laying in the hospital bed, the doctor came in to see how her pain was. I was arguing about the medication the nurse gave her as it was not working and that she needed something else. As Asia was lying there listening, he said she is going to die. My little Asia busted out in tears and said "mama I don't want to die". I wondered why he would say that in front of her, did he not think she would understand what he said. My husband was outside at the car at this time. He was having a hard day dealing with Asia's pain and he too suffered from Post Traumatic Stress disorder from the Vietnam War. As I mentioned earlier it was really hard for him to sit in the hospital room seeing kids crying. He would say he could feel death and the situation of the kids being sick brought back flash backs of him seeing children killed. Seeing his own baby girl Asia in pain was taking a toll on us all and I often wondered if he would explode. I saw the pressure build up many times and it was a good thing he was in the car because if he had heard the doctor say that Asia was going to die in front of her it would have been an ugly situation. Post Traumatic Stress Vietnam veteran's symptoms are not very pretty as my husband probably would have lost it that day. as he was already walking on the edge. My husband had presented to the doctor earlier a letter about his medical condition, I often wondered if the doctor really understood the diagnosis post traumatic stress disorder. There were many days that he sat and stayed in the hospital room and I could see how it was affecting him. The situation was bad because losing everything you have did not help the disorder at all. It made it worse and there were so many days and nights that we were deranged, the stress level was unbelievable. The only good thing that made us hang on was looking in our little girls faces and knowing that they needed and depended on us. We were there only hope. The doctor then prescribed Oxycodone and morphine for breakthrough pain. After we got home, I mentioned to my husband what the doctor said in front of Asia. I could see a fuse being blown; he was already under a great deal of stress. He said when we go back to the hospital he would be having a conversation with the doctor. The medication helped for a very short time as she seemed to become immune to it. When we carried her in for her outpatient visit we explained to them that the medication wasn't working. Asia was crying and refused to walk or even get out of her stroller. Dad told the nurse that he needed to talk with the doctor and of course the nurse knew what it was about, she was in the room when the doctor said that Asia was going to die. The look on the nurse's face showed she knew this was not going to be good. As my husband waited for the doctor they told us we could come into a room. As we entered, there was a social worker, the nurse, and the doctor. Dad asked why were all of them in the room. He told them if it was something he wanted to do to the doctor, no one could prevent it. He then questioned the doctor and of course the doctor apologized, but that was implanted in my child's head and I knew I'm sorry would not be good enough. Asia was too smart and too bright to be fooled. I tried to tell her that the doctor does not have her life in his hands. My husband told the doctor that he needed to find a way to insure Asia that he would be doing everything he could to help her, we expected an apology from him to Asia, and we did not care how he handled it but my baby better not be affected by what he said out of his mouth. To this day he has not forgotten the words the doctor said in front of Asia. I talked with one of my local friends that also had a child with cancer and she told me that he did the same thing with her child. Her child was older than mine and she too had to call him to the side and tell him to never say that again in front of her child. The doctor apologized, but I felt the damage had already been done and that was something you should never tell a child, making them feel you have given up on them.

After that was over the doctor told us that she would now have to be put on the morphine pump because she was in great pain. She could not stand for anyone to touch her body. She told me she had to go to the bathroom but when I went to assist her she began to cry and said "mama please don't move me". I could hardly stand it. I was so deranged seeing her calling for help being in so much pain. They began to attach the morphine pump to her line as we were waiting for her pain to stop she continued to cry. I then told the doctor that the dosage of medication that she was receiving wasn't working because she wasn't being relieved of her pain. He went on to say that it was the right dosage and as it get into her system she would get better. We waited for a while and she was still in great pain. I told the doctor again that the medication wasn't working and if you don't know how to get her out of pain I suggested he call Sloan Kettering hospital. They always seemed to assist my child the correct way. By this time dad and I were getting ugly and the pressure was rising. The doctor said that he felt the dosage was still accurate. I reminded him that Asia requires more pain medication than the average child. I sensed that the doctor did not like taking instructions from the other hospital that has a pain management team. All this time Asia was still sitting in her stroller because she couldn't stand to be touched or moved, the doctor is still telling me that her pain would get better. It was later in the day as we were there all day and it was time for us to leave the clinic I told the doctor that if you really think she'd get better then stay here until we put her in the car to see how much better she'd get. He stayed as we strolled her to the car. She screamed and cried as we tried to put her in the vehicle. I could of died right there as my cup had runneth over and I was about to loose it. I looked at the doctor and I said "you call this pain under control?' He turned red in the face and we left with the pump and breakthrough medication. He did not call the doctor in New York while we were there to inquire about any recommendations to manage her pain. The next day he told me that I was right about the dosage and that she did need a heavier dosage of pain medication so they increased the dosage. Also now the hospice nurse had been contacted and would be coming to the home to monitor the pump and take her blood samples because it was to hard to transport her. The doctor wanted her to be hospitalized and I replied no because I saw how they were about getting her out of pain and I told them that if she needed to be hospitalized I would prefer Sloan Kettering. We of course called Sloan Kettering to inquire as to whether they had received a call from

Merlon Blizzard

our local hospital inquiring about pain management for Asia. I was told they had not received any call. The doctor there told us he would contact our local doctor and discuss it.

Losing Everything

By now we have a foreclosure on our home and had to rent a place to say in between all of these hospital visits and traveling. The credit cards were still being used and resources were little to none. We had moving expenses that we didn't have money for and the bill collectors steadily calling. The telephone calls were getting uglier and uglier. They told my husband that they needed the money and would not be able to work out any plans with us. The fire in our lives seemed to get hotter and hotter. The pressure got so hot with one telephone conversation that I heard my husband tell the bill collector to "kiss his ass". The house was rocking, but our whole world was rocking, marriage and all. You begin to realize that the world can be real cold and there are few that stay in the fire with you. I had asked for donated leave from my job, it seemed if you are not known by someone you would only received little to none but every little bit helped. A few people helped but it was only so much they could give and that was because someone interceded for me.

The hospice nurse was now coming two to three times a week and Asia's blood and platelets were diminishing more frequently, her legs and feet began to swell as fluid increased into her legs and feet. She now had to be cauterized, due to her stomach swelling, her urine wasn't flowing and the catheter had to stay in. Morphine has many side effects, such as constipation and will cause cardiac arrest as well. The whole time I was glad to see Asia getting relief from pain but I was also paying very close attention to the side effects. As the doctor was hooking Asia up to the morphine pump, the nurse called me and her father in a room and informed us that Asia may have a cardiac arrest. This didn't make things any better. I explained to the hospice nurse that I did not want Asia to sleep all the time and she replied if she sleeps too much that she could be given Ritalin but I was very much aware of the side effects of medication and I would prefer that Ritalin not be used. Asia had a strong system when it came to medication, it would take a lot to put her down. She could still respond and talk to you the on the morphine pump. I prayed and asked God to please let my child keep her mind and also let me be present if he had to come and get her, as Asia always wanted me close to her and I needed to be close to her as well. We never left Asia alone as we always made sure someone was close by that was in the family. The doctor in New York even asked us how we went to the bathroom, as we always stayed very close together. Love will do that.

Even though the nurse was there Asia still would not let her do certain things and would let her know that she preferred me to do it. She did not want the nurses at any time to give her a bath or assist her in diaper changes as when Asia first started taking chemotherapy she was potty trained but of course chemotherapy did at one point cause her to go back to diapers as the doctor said with young children it does happen but she didn't stay in diapers the whole time.

As Asia was lying in bed with her feet and legs continuing to swell I knew that fluid was building up in my little girl's body and she was beginning to need oxygen to assist her with her breathing. At first she told the medics that came to set the oxygen up to leave but after she tried it I think she begin to feel it was helping her. Her breathing was becoming shallow and the oxygen machine was so loud. In between the hospice nurse visits they would call to check on Asia and inform us of her blood work results and the nurse was speaking with dad and told him that according to her last labs that were drawn she was going quickly. I saw a look on my husbands face that let me know she said something to him that I really did not want to hear. He began to get angry as the nurse was talking to him as he did not care for the hospice nurse as he said the word hospice meant death.

One Last Hug

On March 10, 2002 we all slept in the same room with Asia and as I was trying to get ready for bed Asia said to me "mama come on and get in the bed with me" and I said ok baby I am coming. I am trying to get all of your medications prepared before I lay down. She waited a little while and said to me again "mama I am waiting for you to get in the bed with me" as I slept with Asia every night and she would wait for me too. If she would awaken and I had left the room she would scream and hollow and say "mama I asked you not to leave me". She would ask me also to hold her hand at night and we would fall to sleep holding hands. I would say to Asia every night "Asia mama loves you" and she would say "I love you too" and this was done every night on a regular basis. She told me one night she said "mama when you hold my hand the devil does not bother me but when we don't hold hands he tries to talk to me". She awakened one night and said that the devil told her to tell me that if I pray for her again that he will never leave her alone. I told her not to believe that and he was trying to scare her but we would continue to pray and he will never have her. I then layed down beside Asia and she told me to get real close so I scooted over real close as our foreheads touched and I asked her if I was close enough and she said yes. So we both drifted off to sleep as I was keeping an eye on her on a real close basis. Asia continued to wake up frequently during the night and would ask Dad to pull her up on the pillow as she would slip down and she could breathe better propped up. As he assisted her he would ask her if her position was ok and she would say yes that it was ok. Dad lying on the left side, I on the right and Chassity to the right of me, we were all together. Dad sleeps light anyway since coming home from Vietnam and has never slept heavy or all night due to his experiences in the war and was constantly on alert. Asia asked dad several times to readjust her position during the night. Dad was laying there listening to her breathing as he said it hurted him so bad to see his baby girl struggle for breath. He told me he asked God to take him instead of her as he felt she had not lived a long life and he had been here for a while. He felt it was so unfair for her to go through the sickness that she had.

As morning came Chassity began getting ready for school, it was the day for the hospice nurse to come. Later on in the middle of the day Dad left to go to the bank and while they were gone I stayed

close to Asia. I thought about taking a shower but did not feel easy
about leaving Asia for over ten minutes at a time. I went toward
the shower but heard a voice speak to me and say "stay close to the
room". I decided not to take the shower at that time and went back
to the room with Asia. I would lie down beside Asia in the bed and
watch TV and talk to her. I would ask her every so often if she was in
pain. I then got up again and thought about taking a quick shower
and as I went toward the bathroom the same voice spoke to me again
saying "stay close to the room". I decided I would give Asia her
bath instead. I filled a pail with water and got her soap and towels
necessary and told her Asia mama is going to give you your bath
now and she said ok. I began to wash her legs and feet carefully and
she just looked at me as I was wiping her legs and I asked her about
her pain. She said she was ok right now. I asked her this because
at one point she could not stand to be touched. As I continued to
wash her legs I noticed I could lift her legs and it was not hurting
her, I said "Asia I can lift your legs and she continued to look at me
as I moved right along continuing to bath her. I noticed once again
I could lift her arm, and I said "Asia look, I can lift your arms". It
was amazing and I began to feel like my Asia's health had taken a
turn for the good. I then proceeded to wash her other arm and I
could move it as well and she did not say anything about it hurting.
I then told her that I was going to change her shirt, she said ok. I

noticed her body was movable so I lifted her back to put my arms
under her and I hugged her and held her in my arms. I said "Asia I
can hold my baby again" and I laid her back down looking her in her
face with this big smile of joy on my face as our eyes locked. I then
realized my Asia had stopped breathing and my mind was completely
blown. Strangely enough the door bell rang and it was the nurse.
How amazing was the timing. I went to the door to let her in and
screaming "Asia has stopped breathing." The nurse told me to call
911. She began mouth to mouth resuscitation. I think my brain
was completely in shock and I was torn to pieces. All I could think
was my baby was gone. The paramedics began working on her but
decided she needed to be taken to the hospital. I had been trying
to call my pastor earlier to tell him that Asia was not doing well. I
was having a hard time reaching him but strangely enough he called
me right after the nurse came in the door. He told me he was on
his way. She had to be taken to the hospital so I called him back to
tell him that we were on our way to the hospital. After calling the
ambulance I called dad and told him that Asia had stopped breathing
and to meet us at the hospital. I didn't know all what I was saying
because I was not expecting Asia to leave me on this day. On the way
to the hospital I was praying in between the calling my mother to tell
her what was going on. After arriving to the emergency room they
continued to try to resuscitate her but she was not responding. The

doctors told us she was gone. By this time Chassity had arrived from school as the hospice nurse was leaving the house she saw Chassity coming home from school and told her that her sister had to be taken to the hospital. Chassity told me she knew something was wrong when she walked in the emergency room and she fell in the Pastors arms and just cried. The Pastor went on to try and comfort Chassity and told me that Chassity did not want to see her sister dead. I told him to let me talk to her and I explained to her that she just look like she is sleep. We stayed there for a little while; I did not want to leave my child in that hospital. I wanted to bring her back home with me. Watching your child die is the most devastating thing in life that a parent can endure. It's so devastating and life changing as well. When we walked out of the hospital room I felt so alone, just like a tree, one of my limbs was cut off. The hollow spot was so great and I knew I had to go home without my child and live without her. While riding in the car I tried to call some relatives and friends to let them know Asia had left us. Two of the people I called were mothers of children who also had kids with the same illness. They cried along with me on the telephone as they too would have to go down the same road. You know it's something about reality that will really open your eyes. I later asked them both if they were going to tell their kids that Asia had gone, and they both said yes. I thought it was best for them to make their own decisions wondering what they were thinking since they both had kids with Neuroblastoma. One of

my friends told her daughter, who was the mother of the older child;

she decided she wanted to come to the funeral. The other friend

said she was going to tell her son because he would be looking for

her and wondering why he hadn't seen her along with his other sick

friends. She said she told him that Asia went to a place where she will

never have to worry about being sick anymore. She would be happy.

She said he thought about it for a few minutes and told her that he

wanted to go with Asia. That same little boy went to Sloan Kettering

in New York shortly after Asia's death for treatment and his mother

called me to tell me that he sat up in the bed and told her he had just

saw Asia. She said she asked him where did he see her at. He told

her she was up in the sky with all of his other friends and they were

having lots of fun. She then said he looked at her and said "Mama I

don't want to take anymore treatment, I want to go with Asia and my

friends". Now this will really make you think. Our kids knew each

other and as they were diagnosed the same year they all left the same

year in the same order. We were like family as we traveled, suffered

and stayed at the same hospitals and the Ronald McDonald House.

Now I can't believe I have to make arrangements for a funeral

for my own child. It felt as though this wasn't happening. But it was

and there was no running place to hide. Now the house filled with

people and there are parts of us that are numb. I constantly felt like
I needed to go and help Asia. We were all in a lost state. The next
morning the Pastor and Asia's god mother came over to help dad and
I make arrangements for Asia. Even though we were doing this it still
felt like I could not believe our Asia was not with us. We went on to
try to prepare her ceremony while still in a state of shock. I got up
the next day looking for one of my credit cards to take to the funeral
home and could not find it. We thought the kids were insured but
discovered the insurance company did not write them on as riders.
While searching for it I became more torn to pieces. I was also taking
her clothes there for them to dress her in. She was dressed in a pink
dress, a white and pink hat, Dora panties, a slip, white stockings and
a pair of little white gloves. She had a toy named Mr. Bucket that ran
by batteries, which happened to come on and began to move across
the floor. Dad and I just looked as the toy continued to run, my
husband said to me "Asia is trying to tell you it's going to be alright"
and afterwards the toy stopped. I know a lot of people may think
this to be strange but this really happened. It did not scare us as it
was a peaceful feeling as this was occurring. We then left to go to the
funeral home.

On the day of Asia's home going services I tried to listen to the
Pastor's message because I needed all the encouragement and strength

that I could receive but I was there and not there at the same time.

I believe I was still in shock. I remember the Pastor saying that

we were given an angel and God does not entrust everybody with

his angels. God foresaw that we would take care of her and knew

how to care for her and that we were the parents selected for this

child. He also said God came back for her because she was pure

and the evilness of this world had not yet infested her so he decided

to take her while she was still pure. He said her trip to Disney was

wonderful but nothing like the trip she is on now. I often think of

what Asia is doing up there with God. He went on to say Isaiah

11:6, that a little child shall lead them. With this said Asia had lead

many people today to church to acknowledge God, because for her

to be so little, she had touched more lives in six years than many of

us whom are forty, fifty or more. Asia also told me that she was not

going to work a job and I said then how are you planning on taking

care of yourself when you grow up and she said "mama I will not be

working a job". I told the Pastor that she had spoken this to me and

he said that she had already taken a good look around and saw how

her parents were surviving and noticed that most people go to work

everyday and that she saw life did not look exciting to her. At her

funeral he said that he believed that God showed her a choice that she

could choose to stay here and deal with the world sickness and other

unhappiness and then he showed her what he had to offer which was complete happiness with no pain. He believed she told him "let's go." Something to think about isn't it? I believe sickness can bring you to a place that you will choose to leave this life.

After the pastor finished the ceremony, I went up to kiss my Asia one more time but it was as if I could feel her knowing I was there. Dad looked at her and put a stuffed toy horse and a book bag that she wanted in with her that she had been waiting for to arrive in the mail in the coffin. Chassity kissed her as well. After that Dad walked out because it was all he could take. It was now time to proceed to the gravesite and I did not want to walk away and leave her there but at the same time I could not stand there to watch them lower her down.

Now its time to go home and reality begins to sink in more and more. I had problems sleeping and the loss seemed to feel greater and greater. All of us were hurting and I wanted to just give up. I begin to wish God had just taken us all. Chassity was alone and never wanted to be an only child as this was the sibling she had prayed and asked God for. Afterwards I was at home one day alone and I hollowed, screamed and cried telling God I want my child back and asking him to help me because this I couldn't do without him. I said to God I will never make it. This is when I realized I was no longer carrying myself but it was God that was carrying me. A light came on and the

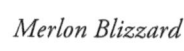

gift of wisdom became so awesome that it is explicable.

As the following Sunday came and Chassity came into my bedroom and asked me "mama are we going to church"? I said " Chassity I don't think I am going." I was feeling really depressed and grieving badly. She same over to where I was lying and flipped the covers back and said "mama yes you are going, it is where you need to be". . It was such a task for me just to dress myself. I needed God to help me put my shoes on. I looked at Chassity and realized I was reaping what I had sown into her. Proverbs 22:6 Train up a child in the way he should go; and when he is old, he will not depart from it. It was her and my husband that gave me the will to hold on because I knew we needed each other. I knew Chassity still needed her mother. I learned to take one minute at a time instead of one day at the time and that I was not the driver but the rider in this life's journey. Dad being a Post Traumatic Stress victim I often wondered if he would kill himself as some parents did commit suicide.

Now that Asia was gone it continued to get worse, as we had to move again and we had little to no money. This time we put our household furnishings in storage and lived with some friends until we could finance somewhere to go. It seemed each move brought us to less and less house. This was hard trying to live around people while you are grieving. I did not return to work right away as it was difficult for me. I know we needed money but keeping my mind was a job in itself. A lot of our clothes that we wore were riding around with us in our vehicle. People think you can just move on after the funeral but it seemed it just got worse. I remember Chassity telling me one day "mama I don't feel like this is getting any better" and I heard the same comment from Dad. I don't think you ever get over losing your child, you just learn to live with it which is a hollow spot and pain. It's called the missing link. There is no cure and nothing fills the void. Somedays you may be able to talk about it and sometimes you don't want to discuss it. Seems time moves so slowly for the healing process and there are trigger points that you have to deal with that remind you of the pain and loss. As we are still in debt today and have not recovered financially I do not regret anything I did that was in reference to saving my child's life. I used the credit cards for our life threatening needed situations which I feel is what credit cards are for (emergencies) and catastrophic situations. Grief is not the same for everybody and everyone grieves differently. Some days you may do fine and some times you can be just driving down the street and just burst out crying. There are no days that go by and you don't think of them. Every child has a place and no one can fill the place but the person the place was made for.

Dreams

Asia shared many of her dreams with me and talked to me about seeing angels and evil forces. One morning I was going to work (when Asia was in remission) and Asia came running in the bathroom, telling me she saw an evil person sitting beside Chassity in the bed. I went back to the bedroom with her and she pointed to where she saw it at. Chassity then got up and said "why was it sitting beside me"? Then there was an incident when we went to New York at the Ronald McDonald House and Chassity said she woke up and Asia was sitting on the bed whispering to someone but could not see anybody. She asked Asia who was she taking to and she said Asia jumped on her playing in a way and never answered her. My husband said that sometimes at night he could feel children's presents in the Ronald McDonald House. A lot of children have passed away that were receiving treatment that stayed at the Ronald McDonald House. As we were returning from one of Asia's all day hospital treatment visits, dad was strolling Asia to our room at the Ronald

McDonald House and Asia told him to look at the head that was in the plant, and he asked where was it but no one could see it but her. She was never frightened by any of this. Asia also shared a dream with me which she saw a lot of angels were dressed in black robes. They were not good angels and they were after her but then Jesus appeared, and threw her a sword and afterwards they all disappeared. She said Jesus told her whenever evil forces came to her to use her sword. She would speak words of wisdom to been so little. Dad would ask her who was she and where did she come from? She would look at him but never answered. When Asia was in pain she ask me to play a scripture healing tape. She would lie there listening to the prayers. She too would reach for my hand and ask me to pray for her.

There are times when I feel like I can feel her because I knew only her body went to the grave but her spirit is very much alive. I began to have many dreams about Asia as she left this side of life. I believe it was her way, as well as God's way, to help me with my grief...

Asia left this life March 11, 2002 and I had a dream on April 9, 2002 that Asia was at the hospital in a hospital gown and she said to me "mama all the tumors in my legs are gone and my bone marrow is clean. I hugged her and said "my baby is healed." April 2002 Chassity had a dream that Asia came into her bedroom and sat on the side of the bed. She asked Asia if she remembered what happened here and Asia nodded her head yes and smiled. Chassity said Asia looked very pretty. April 19, 2002 I dreamed I saw two bright balls glittering with light that represented Asia. I then dreamed again that Asia was asleep and I told her that I needed to change her panties, I looked and she still had on the same Dora panties that she left here wearing. I believe she was telling me that she knew I had put those Dora panties on her. Again in the same month I dreamed crocodiles were trying to get me and I tried to push them back with a stick but another animal appeared which looked like a turtle shell and when I tried to push it back with a stick, a lot of butterflies came out of his back. I received a mother's day card the next day with a butterfly cut out inside the card and I went to pick Chassity up from school and she had a butterfly print on her shirt. I told Chassity about my dream and I said I believe those butterflies mean something and she said" I believe God is telling you "Asia has her wings." May 22, 2002 I dreamed Asia was laying in her coffin on her side and I went up to awaken her and she said "mama I was not sleep, I was just resting and I am alright". She said "my legs don't hurt anymore", and she was dressed in an angel outfit and had a head full of hair. That same month I dreamed that Asia came to me and said "mama whenever you feel you miss me, look into my pictures and there I will be." I could actually see her move and look back at me. July 2, 2002 I

dreamed I saw Asia was sitting in her stroller nodding in and out of sleep, she looked up at me and said "mama I saw your name written in the book of life and it is written in very big letters," she then smiled and said "mama I see mine too". December 2002 I dreamed of my grandfather who died before Asia and Chassity was born and he said to me" I know you are sad because of your baby, but your connection with her did not stop, the connection continues on." He said he saw Asia and my baby sister Shirlette when they went up. He also asked if Chassity told me. I thought my grandfather must be watching over us. December 2002 I dreamed Asia was lying in my lap with a T-shirt on and asked me if I remembered when I use to ask you to hold my hand and I said yes and she then reached to hold my hand and held my finger. February 2003 Chassity dreamed Asia came down from the heavens on an elevator that was operated by Moses, Asia said she came to visit but she had to go back. Chassity asked Asia who lets you come to visit us, "and Asia said God does". March 2003 I dreamed Asia had grown some and was looking healthy. She walked to me and hugged me. I said to her "Asia I really do miss you and she said "mama I came to earth to do what I had to do. I had to leave and you too will have to do the same and afterwards you too will leave". Her hair was combed with a ponytail on each side of her head. In the dream she could feel I was missing her and knew I needed to be comforted. May 2003 I dreamed Asia and I were lying in the bed together and she said "mama I know you have been moving around but since you are back in a house now we can sleep together again". I also dreamed that Asia had been gone for a while and I was wondering where she was and she appeared. I said to her "I am so surprised to see that you are handling things all grown up" and she smiled but we knew we were separated and that she could not stay. She let me know that she was ok and although I wasn't on her side of life, she was doing ok. She had a big smile on her face when she appeared to me. June 2005 I dreamed Asia was rubbing my face with her hands and when I woke up Oliver (the cat) was rubbing my jaw with his paw.

The dreams have continued until this day and I keep a journal and write them down. I look at the time frame of my dreams; the dreams appeared more frequently at first .It's as though she knows I miss her so much that she tries to help me. I guess she has things to attend to in heaven. As time has moved on I have dreamed of her being a little bigger, it's as if she is still growing. True love goes beyond the grave or death. I too believe because we are spiritually connected that is why I have the dreams and feelings that I do.

As I said earlier the other two family's kids followed after Asia in March, the little boy in November and the girl in December 2002.

I and Dad attended all of three kid's funerals in one year and each funeral took us back to our daughter. The mother that helped me with information about the New York hospital daughter also died the same year. We couldn't make her funeral as it was right behind Asia's and I could not stand to see another little girl lying in a coffin. She lived a little farther than the others from us. The day she died my husband called me saying two butterflies flew up to him and then flew off together. I later heard her mother had a little girl and named her with my child and her daughters names combined. Just think when we see our children again it will never be another good-bye but a forever hello.

I wonder why children are not tested for Neuroblastoma at birth and throughout age three since this is the age most known for the cancer to occur. I have been told that there are some mothers who have found out during their pregnancy that their child has Neuroblastoma. The earlier this disease is diagnosed the better the chances for survival.

Chassity's Story

In school, Chassity wrote a brief story about her beloved sister. It is titled My own Personal Angel.

"Can you believe that I actually had a little angel for a short period of time? The little angel's name was Asia. Her birthday is November 4, 1995. Her treatment took place at Memorial Sloan Kettering hospital in New York and some at the Children's Hospital of the Kings Daughters in Virginia, causing us to travel back and forth. All of here treatment was very aggressive, but what do you expect when someone is fighting a life threatening illness. During our traveling the seasons changed all of the time from summer to fall, winter so spring and then summer again. While my sister was going through treatment, I felt devastated for her because she had to go through a lot. She lost her hair, eyebrows and her fingers turned light brown from the medication that she had to be treated with. Well anyway the type of cancer my sister had was Neuroblastoma. This cancer is the most devastating and aggressive cancer you can ever

have. When she was around three years old we saw signs of limping so we had to have her checked out by a doctor. Then afterwards we found out she had cancer and was immediately hospitalized. Then Asia went into remission for a little over a year and then the cancer came back returning twice as aggressive, she went back through treatment again. While we thought she was going to beat the odds against this devastating cancer, God had other plans.

My sister and I were very close and we slept in the same bed for six years until one day she departed from our family on March 11, 2002, so we thought. Her last words were "Where is Chassity? My mother said "at school" and where is my daddy? And my mom replied he is on his way home and she did not say anything else after that. She left to be a supernatural Angel. I will miss her and that will never change. I will always miss her soft hands, her sweet spirit, and her firey side and finally I will miss her on the other side of my bed.

This experience was meaningful and life changing to me because we should always take time with our love ones. You may not always have as much time as you think to spend with your love ones and you should always tell them that you love them. You should never mistreat them in any way because you will pay for it later on down the road. See what a lot of people don't know is Asia was an A.O.L. What that means was an

Angel on Loan. Now I am going to leave you with that thought."

-Chassity M. Blizzard.

I often think if Asia could speak to any of us today she would say "If you could see me now, I'm walking the streets of gold, If you could see me now, I'm standing strong and whole, If you could see me now, you'd know I've seen his face, If you could see me now, you'd know the pain is erased. You wouldn't want me to ever leave this place, if you could see me now".

She never once complained and was a true soldier.

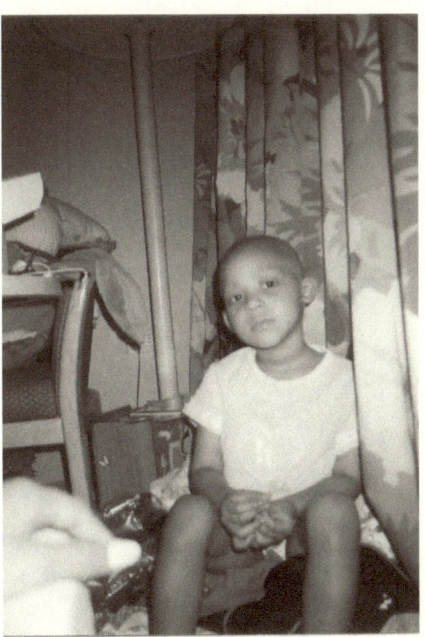

Should you happen to walk this road or are walking this road please check out the following organizations for help and assistance.

Merlon Blizzard

Also please contact the social worker upon the hospital you are receiving treatment. Should you decide to make donations to a society, please remember Neuroblastoma cancer as it is rare and yet children are dying everyday and parents needs a lot of assistance.

Recommended References:

www.speciallove.org

Cancer Care

Edmarc Hospice for Children

American Cancer Society

www. candlelighters.org

www. Caringbridge.org

Make a Wish Foundation

N-Blastoma @ listserv.acor.org